A PRACTICAL INTRODUCTION
TO MENTAL HEALTH ETHICS

As a mental health nurse, possessing an ethical sensibility and developing ethical reasoning is vital. This book is a practical introduction to the skills and knowledge the mental health nurse is professionally required to develop in their journey towards effectively managing complex ethical decisions. Written with the training mental health nurse in mind, this book is a clear and concise guide on how to approach common, ethically-complex situations mental health nurses will eventually find themselves faced with. It includes textboxes that take the reader into a 'real world' scenario to help them explore the moral and ethical issues discussed throughout the chapter.

To ensure professional currency, the content of this book is mapped to the Nursing and Midwifery Council's pre-registration education standards of 2010, and uses a scenario-based approach in order to provide a pragmatic and robust resource.

A Practical Introduction to Mental Health Ethics is essential reading for pre-registration mental health nursing students, while also being of value to registered mental health nurses working in ethically challenged areas such as dementia care, psychiatric intensive care units.

Grahame Smith is the subject head of Allied Health in the Faculty of Education, Health and Community, Liverpool John Moores University, Henry Cotton Campus, UK. He is an experienced mental health nurse who has worked in a variety of mental health service settings.

A PRACTICAL INTRODUCTION TO MENTAL HEALTH ETHICS

Grahame Smith

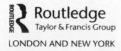

Routledge
Taylor & Francis Group

LONDON AND NEW YORK

First published 2017
by Routledge
2 Park Square, Milton Park, Abingdon, Oxon OX14 4RN

and by Routledge
711 Third Avenue, New York, NY 10017

Routledge is an imprint of the Taylor & Francis Group, an informa business

British Library Cataloguing-in-Publication Data
A catalogue record for this book is available from the British Library

Library of Congress Cataloging in Publication Data
Names: Smith, Grahame, author. Title: A practical introduction to mental
health ethics / Grahame Smith. Description: Abingdon, Oxon ; New York,
NY : Routledge, 2017. | Includes bibliographical references and index.
Identifiers: LCCN 2016027107| ISBN 9781138840270 (hardback : alk.
paper) | ISBN 9781138840300 (paperback : alk. paper) | ISBN 9781315732886
(ebook)Subjects: | MESH: Psychiatric Nursing--ethicsClassification:
LCC RC455.2.E8 | NLM WY 160 | DDC 174.2/96890231--dc23LC
record available at https://lccn.loc.gov/2016027107

ISBN: 978-1-138-84027-0 (hbk)
ISBN: 978-1-138-84030-0 (pbk)
ISBN: 978-1-315-73288-6 (ebk)

Typeset in Bembo
by Fish Books Ltd.

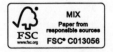

Printed and bound in Great Britain by
TJ International Ltd, Padstow, Cornwall

CONTENTS

INTRODUCTION

Overview of the book

I hope you will find this book useful, it has been written with the pre-registration mental health nursing student in mind, however aspects of the book will be just as useful to other healthcare students and practitioners.

The idea for this book arose from my interest in mental health ethics and more importantly my teaching practice. For some students ethics appears to be a subject that is esoteric and quite difficult to make sense of especially when thinking about their everyday practice. My intention was to write a book that is accessible to all, and a stepping stone to considering the subject in more depth. I also wanted to make the book pragmatic (Brendel 2006) by considering:

- the practical nature of ethical inquiry;
- the multi-faceted nature of ethics;
- the role of the individual perspective; and
- that knowledge changes and evolves.

This is why I have focused on the development of effective ethical reasoning within a clinical context, and suggested a pragmatic framework to undertake this skill:

1 Recognise the ethical issues.
2 Gather the facts and values.
3 Consider the rules.
4 Look at any underpinning moral theories.
5 Consider all options.
6 Make a decision and test it.
7 Act and reflect on the outcome.

In addition the nurse has to pay attention to the unique nature of mental health care, the twin issues of power and control, in essence making sense of the values inherent within a given situation. Paying attention to the values inherent within a situation is part of the ethical reasoning process, rather than re-invent the wheel this book identifies how this process interfaces with another process called values-based practice. Considering values requires the student to:

1 Acknowledge the service user's perspective.
2 Take a balanced approach and ensure the service user's values are considered.
3 Truly listen to the service user's story.
4 Make sure this story is fully represented.

Sometimes students struggle to ethically reason due to not being able to identify what an ethical issue is. This may be due in part to not recognising the ethical dimension of our practice. There is an ethical dimension to everything we do as nurses, when to make decisions and then when to act and intervene. This also includes the acts we do in everyday life:

> All of us must make ethical choices. Sometimes those choices seem so easy that we do not see them as choices. We don't consciously decide to comfort a close friend whose son was just killed; we just do.
>
> *(LaFollette 2007: 7)*

How to use the book

This book has been predominantly written for students who are on a pre-registration mental health nursing programme. On this basis this book is underpinned by the Standards for Pre-registration Nursing Education of the Nursing and Midwifery Council (NMC). These standards aim to:

> enable nurses to give and support high quality care in rapidly changing environments. They reflect how future services are likely to be delivered, acknowledge future public health priorities and address the challenges of long-term conditions, an ageing population, and providing more care outside hospitals. Nurses must be equipped to lead, delegate, supervise and challenge other nurses and healthcare professionals. They must be able to develop practice, and promote and sustain change. As graduates they must be able to think analytically, use problem-solving approaches and evidence in decision-making, keep up with technical advances and meet future expectations.
>
> *(NMC 2010: 4–5)*

In addition to this aim, by the end of their programme the student will be expected to be competent, possessing the professionally required knowledge and skills

(NMC 2010; Smith and Rylance 2016). These expectations or requirements are articulated in a framework or domains, there are four domains for each field:

- professional values;
- communication and interpersonal skills;
- nursing practice and decision-making; and
- leadership, management and team working.

Each domain is underpinned by a number of corresponding statements which indicate the professional competencies the student is expected to achieve by end of their training. These statements use the term 'must' throughout, a normative element which gives these statements an ethical dimension. In addition the standards hold the view that student nurses should 'act with professionalism and integrity, and work within agreed professional, ethical and legal frameworks and processes to maintain and improve standards' (NMC 2010: 5).

This expectation of working within the NMC's (2015a) code continues throughout the nurse's post-qualifying life, and a new post-qualifying process called revalidation (NMC 2015b) reinforces this expectation. These professional expectations are reflected throughout the book. It is important to recognise at this juncture that this book is not a substitute for the learning delivered on a pre-qualifying programme, rather it is intended to complement this learning by being an open and accessible learning resource. I would also advocate reading widely; this book is one of the first on mental health ethics aimed at mental health nursing students, however there are a number of good texts available within a number of fields, such as nursing, psychiatry, counselling and psychotherapy. There is also a generic mental health ethics text available, which is edited by Phil Baker and is an excellent background read.

In terms of the structure of the book each chapter is organised in a way that takes the student on a learning journey, from introducing the notion of ethical reasoning to presenting the opportunity for the student to try this out within their supervised practice.

Generally the book can be seen to be divided into two notional parts. Chapters 1–3 tease out the ethical dimension of mental health nursing practice; in addition Chapter 3 explores ethical reasoning and presents a specific ethical reasoning framework. Chapters 4–9 explore this ethical reasoning framework in action by using a consistent scenario approach. The first three chapters also use a scenario approach; however the scenarios are specific to each chapter. Chapter 4 introduces the 'Michael scenario' and then each subsequent chapter corresponds to a stage in the ethical reasoning process.

To promote consistency each chapter will state the aim of the chapter within the first section of the chapter, the background section. As previously stated a scenario approach is used, sometimes the scenario will be further developed within 'text boxes' and on occasion there will be a commentary on the scenario within the main body of the text. Using a scenario approach provides the student with a clear example of how their learning can be applied to practice. This approach is not exclusive; certainly it is expected that the student will apply learning from their own experiences to test the knowledge contained within each chapter. The student may find during this process that they do not agree with a given approach, which is fine: be critical, but also support your views by engaging in further research. At the end of each chapter, the chapter will be summarised through a 'key learning point' section, this will give the student the opportunity to reflect on their learning.

To be consistent the term service user is used throughout the book. The term nurse is also used; the term nurse captures a number of fields of practice beyond mental health nursing. These fields of practice will also manage people who are mentally distressed, so where the term nurse is used it generally relates to nursing people in mental health distress, and where the specific term mental health nurse is used this relates specifically to the mental health nursing field.

Chapter overview

Chapter 1 focuses on the ethical dimension of the clinical decision-making process. Nurses as busy practitioners have a tendency to think that ethical reasoning is divorced from every day practice, almost a hidden dimension. So this chapter teases out the notion that everyday practice also has an ethical dimension. Once the nurse recognises this ethical dimension they can then engage effectively with ethical reasoning as a systematic process.

Chapter 2 in some ways is similar to Chapter 9, in that it explores the notion of expert practice; however it focuses on the ethical aspect of expert practice which includes the development of the ethical self. This is the self that the mental health nurse will use as a key part of developing and maintaining therapeutic relationships. Working in these relationships requires the mental health nurse to pay attention to the evidence-base, coupled with being emotionally sensitive.

Chapter 3 starts to introduce ethical reasoning as way to resolve ethical challenges. This type of reasoning is not something that only nurses do; it is something we all do, something that starts in childhood. The chapter presents a balanced approach, one that considers the values inherent within a given situation while recognising that mental health nursing can be fast paced and complex.

Chapter 4 presents the first step in the ethical reasoning process, recognising ethical issues. On this basis there is a focus on considering the role of ethical distress and ethical sensitivity. This is contextualised by the unique nature of mental health nursing practice especially around consent and capacity.

Chapter 5 looks at how the mental health nurse gathers facts and values as part of the second stage in the ethical reasoning process. Nurses might assume that a 'fact is a fact' when it may be a 'value turned into a fact' through a process such as the assessment process. Gathering information via the assessment process can lead to ethical conflict especially if the service user's viewpoint is lost in the language of this process.

Chapter 6 is the third stage in the ethical reasoning process focusing on the use of rules, legal and professional frameworks, policies and clinical guidelines. The rule-based frameworks are there to guide the mental health nurse, they are not all-encompassing and they are not specific to every situation a mental health nurse will face in their practice.

Chapter 7 is the fourth stage in the ethical reasoning process and explores a number of major ethical theories that the mental health nurse will find useful when ethically reasoning. These theories relate to duties and outcomes, principles, and character, there is also a focus on how ethical theories can work together in a pragmatic way.

Chapter 8 captures the final stages of the ethical reasoning process considering how the outcomes of an ethical decision can help improve a nurse's future practice. When implementing an agreed outcome the nurse will have explored different options, they will have tested the decision, and on implementation of that decision they will have reflected on their actions. These reflections should lead to learning with a focus on improving their future practice.

Chapter 9, though not a formal part of the book's ethical reasoning process, explores how the development of robust ethical reasoning skills are crucial in relation to the nurse's lifelong learning journey. This includes the professional commitment for mental health nurses to be lifelong learners; this commitment is now being measured through the revalidation process.

When working through each chapter I hope that the underlying message that mental health ethics is a about humanity and healing shines through:

> To be ethical is to be human. If we shirk the challenge of ethics we risk sacrificing our right to be called human.
>
> *(Barker 2011: 26)*

> The human sciences at the beginning of the twenty-first century remain mired in a quiet but serious and abiding conceptual crisis. Nowhere is this crisis more urgent than the area in which I practice, psychiatry, which faces an ongoing ethical challenge to define what it means to be a human subject. … In the rush to understand, explain, and treat with new rapid-fire technologies, many psychiatrists have disengaged from more plodding, uncertain and ambiguous forms of approaching patients, such as insight-orientated psychotherapy and psychoanalysis.
>
> *(Brendel 2006: 1)*

1
CLINICAL DECISION-MAKING WITHIN AN ETHICAL CONTEXT

Background

The aim of this chapter is to explore the ethical dimension of the clinical decisions that mental health nurses make on a daily basis. Mental health nurses may not always recognise that the decisions they make have an ethical dimension. In other words, this dimension tends to be hidden (Smith 2012b). This does not mean mental health nurses are not ethical in their practice, however they may not fully recognise the context they practice within, where 'a fully conscious adult patient of normal intelligence may be treated without consent, not for the protection of others (though this is also possible) but in their own interests' (Fulford 2009: 62).

To act ethically the mental health nurse has to be aware of the context they practice within and they have to ethically reason in a way that is systematic and justifiable. By reasoning in this way the nurse will develop a justifiable position which considers the rules inherent within a situation such as the law, it will also pay attention to the facts and the values, and it will be embedded within a relevant ethical theory (Bloch and Green 2009; Barker 2011). These considerations among others will be developed in more detail as the book progresses. As a starting point lets us consider what ethics are, the historical nature of mental nursing practice, evidence-based practice, and the clinical decision-making process and its relationship to being ethical.

Ethics, 'derived from the Greek ethikos, meaning "disposition", has a philosophical home in the discourse of moral philosophy, the study of conduct with respect to whether an act is right or wrong, to the goodness and badness of the motives and ends of the act' (Bloch and Green 2009: 3). Ethics or ethical theories are divided into normative theories, which focus on 'what actions are right, what ought to be done, what motives are good, and what characteristics are virtuous' (Smith 2012b: 144), and non-normative theories. The latter are descriptive, describing ethical beliefs, conduct, and how people ethically reason (Smith 2012b). This book will concentrate on ethical theories which are normative theories. The importance of understanding what constitutes being ethical is important for the mental health nurse as they will be expected to professionally act ethically and do the right thing (Smith 2012b; NMC 2015a).

On entering your new ward a service user pushes past you, shouting 'I am one with the angels, you devils!' He reaches the ward door and kicks it a few times. He then promptly turns around and goes back to his bed. The staff member at the door tells you not to worry as John knows the door is locked and he is not going anywhere. On reading John's case notes you notice that John is well known to services and he has a diagnosis of schizophrenia. He was admitted to the ward after he stopped taking his medication; he then became aggressive towards his Mum. John would not restart his medication while at home, but he did agree to come into hospital. Once admitted John agreed to restart his medication. You decide to have a chat with John. On entering his room you notice that he has not washed for days. John will not fully engage with you; he just keeps repeating that he wants to go home. You ask one of the staff about John, and they mentioned that he sleeps all day, but there is nothing that can be done as this is his 'human right'. When looking at John's medication card you notice he misses most of the medication that is prescribed in the day.

The historical context

Mental health nursing as a specialist field of practice is a recent phenomenon and one that does not exist within a vacuum (Roberts 2005; Foucault 1961; Porter 2002; Nolan 1993). Mental health nursing in the UK has always been closely aligned with the medical discipline of psychiatry which has largely shaped how mental health nurses practice today (Nolan 1993; Zilboorg and Henry 1941; Fulford *et al.* 2006). The work of Nolan (1993) on the history and development of mental health nursing from the eighteenth century onwards provides a 'template' to better understand this alignment.

Mental health nurses have not always been called mental health nurses and even today there are two titles in common use: mental health nurse and psychiatric nurse. Currently the professionally registered title is 'registered nurse – mental health' (NMC 2010). Historically, mental health nurses have had a number of titles bestowed upon them from the title of keeper then to attendant and then finally to psychiatric nurse or mental health nurse (Nolan 1993: 6–7). All of these titles were used as common titles and with those titles came a variety of roles. The role of the keeper was to look after both the house and the mentally ill that resided within the house, whereas the role of the attendant was to look after the institution including controlling the 'inmates' and also to be a servant for the medical staff (ibid.). The role of the attendant was a direct historical development from the role of the keeper, however like the keeper, attendants were still un-trained and there was no common agreement of what a good attendant did besides looking after the institution, training would be given on an ad-hoc basis and dependent on the motivation of the medical superintendent (ibid.). The attendant was generally expected to be a rule keeper, an enforcer of the rules, a servant to the patients, a spiritual guide, and an intermediary between doctor and patient (ibid.: 53–54). Attendants like 'keepers' were also 'prized' for their abilities to do physical work such as cleaning and manual labour (ibid.: 48).

There was a shift to systematically training attendants this happened from 1889 where attendants were now required to attend a national training course and from 1923 female attendants started to be called nurses, however males were still called attendants until 1926 (ibid.). This change from the title of attendant to the title of nurse started to reflect the belief that the 'embryonic' mental health nurse should have a more caring role and, possibly as a consequence, deliver therapy (ibid.). An underpinning influence on the historical development of the mental health nurse role was the burgeoning belief that mental health problems should and could be treated and possibly 'cured' (Clarke 2008). Certainly the advent of the 'mental asylum' from the eighteenth century onwards came into being on the belief the 'mad' could be 'cured' with the right therapy (Jones 1996). At that time the attendant role was in the forefront of delivering this right therapy which was based on good basic care including exercise and good nutrition (ibid.). Over time elements such as 'observation and control' also became part of this therapy and finally during the embryonic development of the mental health nurse role further therapies started to emerge, such as psychiatric medication and psychological interventions (Nolan 1993; Shorter 1997).

This move towards therapy and treatment was ultimately influenced by the medicalisation of madness (Shorter 1997; Read 2004). Historically this medicalisation process meant that madness was described has having different forms, and over time, as psychiatry developed as a medical profession, different psychiatric disorders were identified, as were their accompanying treatments (Berrios 1996; Sims 2003; Oyebode 2008).

This process of describing and identifying psychiatric disorders and their accompanying treatments also led mental health nursing down a similar path in that mental health nursing delivered some of those treatments (Clarke 2008). By the twentieth century, with the discipline of psychiatry becoming truly medicalised and using scientific methods, mental health nursing also followed suit in using more scientific methods (Zilboorg and Henry 1941; Clarke 2008; Gournay 2009).

Contemporary mental health nursing has certainly moved from treating mental health service users in what in hindsight could be seen at times as a brutal and with immoral ways (Clarke 2008). Read (2004) highlights that mental health service users from the seventeenth century onwards were confined and made to conform, and such treatments as bloodletting and fettering were regularly used. Nowadays bloodletting as a mental health treatment would not be allowed; it is not evidence-based, and mental health service users also have rights which are enshrined within statutory law (Read 2004; Clarke 2008). It is important to note that confining and conforming still takes place through the use of implicit and explicit interventions (Coppock and Hopton 2000; Roberts 2005). Explicit interventions include the use of mental health law, restraint, seclusion, locked ward doors, and the administration of medicines (Roberts 2005). Whereas implicit interventions take more subtle forms such as controlling through levels of observation, record keeping, the assessment and care planning process, the delivery of care, and so on (Roberts 2005; Jones and Eales 2009).

Having power to use both implicit and explicit interventions stems from the use of the mental illness concept: even though the use of this concept is conceptually controversial, it does mean that once an individual is labelled mentally ill the mental health nurse may be sanctioned by society to control that individual (Roberts 2004, 2005). Partly this approach emanates from the view that an individual who is labelled mentally ill has an increased potential to exhibit diminished judgement and because of this they are then perceived to be more risky or dangerous than the 'average person' in society (Radden 2002; Smith 2012b). Let us return to the chapter scenario:

> John has a diagnosis of schizophrenia. He is also presenting as a risk towards his mother when he is at home. While on the ward he does not appear to be a risk, and he is taking his medication; or is he? He is willing to stay on the ward by not actively trying to leave the ward; he bangs the ward door, realises it is locked and then returns to his bed. He sleeps all day; is this a problem? It is in terms of him not taking his medication. Is it a human right to sleep all day?
>
> It appears that there are a number of areas of concern regarding John's stay on the ward. What is also concerning is that the mental health nurses on the ward may be unaware of the duty of care they have towards John and implications of using sanctioned power such as a locked door. This lack of awareness may reflect the 'lack of societal will to question the power that mental health services hold' (Smith 2012b: 151), leading to some ethical issues being hidden away.

Evidence-based practice

There is a strong positivist or scientific influence prevalent within contemporary mental health nursing practice similar to the practice of psychiatry (Clarke 2008; Newell and Gournay 2009; DH 2006a, 2006b). This influence can not only be seen to be prevalent it also can be seen to dominant the way mental health practitioners construct their respective practice (DH 2006a, 2006b; NMC 2010). As an example mental health nurses will tend to empirically conceptualise the mental distress of a service user in terms of the service user's diagnosis and subsequent symptomology; in addition clinical guidelines are likely to be catalogued under a diagnosis (Newell and Gournay 2009; Gournay 1995). Returning to the chapter scenario John has a diagnosis of schizophrenia; he has auditory hallucinations and delusions, however he is more than a diagnosis, like everyone else he has hopes and aspirations and should be treated in a person-centred way (Watkins 1998; Smith 2012a).

Evidence-based practice (EBP) is a dominant form of scientific knowledge within mental health nursing practice (Smith 2014). Using this type of knowledge requires the mental nurse to base and justify their clinical decision-making on the best evidence available (ibid.). To ensure the best evidence is available clinical guidelines will be a good source; these guidelines will use evidence which includes the testimonies of clinical experts to the systematic review of Randomised Control Trials (RCTs) (ibid.). The best type of evidence is RCT based evidence, this type of evidence is continually being updated, hence the changes in clinical guidelines (ibid.). On this basis when making clinical decisions (ibid.) mental health nurses should, where possible:

- identify the most appropriate literature;
- critically assess the evidence, considering whether it is reliable and/or valid;
- apply the chosen evidence; and
- evaluate the application of this evidence.

The process above is very similar to the activities of evidence-based medicine, however evidence-based mental health nursing should not neglect the importance of evidence gathered from the mental health nurse-service user relationship (Perraud *et al.* 2006). The scientific approach that underpins mental health practice also extends to the way information is collected about mental health service users. Psychiatrists primarily collect information through a psychiatric examination process, this process is standardised and the information accrued from this process is available to the multi-disciplinary team including the mental health nurse (Fulford *et al.* 2006; Smith 2014). The mental health nurse builds on this information through the use of assessment methods built on a psycho-social approach, which should be reliable and valid (Gournay 2009; Smith 2014).

A good example of the use of a scientific assessment approach within mental health nursing practice is the way mental health nurses currently assess clinical risk (Eales 2009; Rylance and Simpson 2012). To collect clinical risk information a mental health nurse will use an assessment tool which has been designed specifically to collect quantifiable information with the further intention of assisting in the predicting and subsequent management of clinical risk (Rylance and Simpson 2012; Welsh and Lyons 2001). One of the limitations with this approach to assessing risk is that according to Welsh and Lyons (2001: 302) a 'tool developed for research purposes may not address practitioner needs'. Welsh and Lyons (ibid.: 302) provide an example in that 'one off scoring systems' do not and cannot 'reflect the dynamic and often protracted nature of risk behaviour'.

It has to be acknowledged that just using assessment tools to assess risk is not in accordance with best practice (Rylance and Simpson 2012). The mental health nurses should be using a structured risk assessment approach where information is collected through reliable and valid risk assessment tools and then used in conjunction with the nurse's knowledge of the service user and the service user's own views (ibid.). Mental health nurses develop their knowledge and skills or practice knowledge over a number of years, the foundation of this knowledge is based on knowledge from the sciences and from the interpersonal dimension of their practice (Welsh and Lyons 2001; Smith 2012c). This knowledge is further developed into 'ways of knowing'; the work of Carper (1978) identifies four ways of nursing knowing: empiric knowing, aesthetic knowing, personal knowing and ethical knowing. Added to these layers of knowledge and knowing is the nurses own experiences of being a practitioner, which in turn subsequently shapes their practice and their understanding of their practice (Welsh and Lyons 2001; Benner 1982). Experienced nurses understanding their practice as clinical experts means that they have a high level of skills and are using both rational and intuitive knowledge (Benner and Tanner 1987; Hardy et al. 2002).

Knowing intuitively is seen as a common phenomenon, however it is not always valued as scientific knowing (Benner and Tanner 1987; Welsh and Lyons 2001). It is evident that experienced nurses address some clinical problems intuitively especially complex mental health situations where a mental health nurse has to respond immediately, in the aftermath of their actions they will provide an intellectualise rationale, using scientific knowledge to justify their actions (Welsh and Lyons 2001; Hardy et al. 2002). Knowing and acting intuitively links to a form of knowledge which is situational and in turn tacit (Welsh and Lyons 2001; Cutcliffe 1997; Benner and Tanner 1987). This realm of knowledge, which has come to be called 'tacit knowledge', is also known originally via the work of Polanyi (1958) as the 'tacit component of knowledge'. By reflecting on their experiences in a structured way the mental health nurse converts this tacit knowledge into formal knowledge which can be used in similar situations in the future (Welsh and Lyons 2001; Schön 1983). Welsh and Lyons (2001: 304) describe this conversion process of tacit knowledge into formal knowledge as building a virtual 'tacit knowledge store', which is underpinned by the mental health nurse's scientific knowledge. The future use of this store of tacit knowledge is activated by tacit knowing in-action (Schön 1983) and pattern matching (Crook 2001); knowing a situation.

This tacit knowledge is accrued through the nurse knowing the service user, in other words working with the service user's story (Bracken and Thomas 2005). Mental health nurses should be comfortable working in this way especially nurses who are orientated towards using a talking therapy approach (Hurley 2009; Hurley and Rankin 2008). Though the key factor in being effective in working with the client's story is not to interpret a client's story but to work with the client's story in the context of the whole person and not take a segmented approach (Smith 2012a; Bracken and Thomas 2005). By looking at only fragments of the client's story the mental health nurse runs the risk of neutralising the story and in turn the meaning of the story is lost (Bracken and Thomas 2005). This approach fits with the use of a recovery-based approach (Smith 2014). Returning to John, this approach should:

- promote wellbeing;
- maximise opportunity;
- empower John to take control; and
- facilitate and support John in finding meaning and purpose.

Making clinical decisions

Mental health nurses are accountable for their practice decisions. Professionally these decisions have to be person-centred and partnership focused, they also have to be based on the best available evidence, the process should be systematic with agreed outcomes, and where the nurse does have the necessary expertise they should sign-post appropriately (NMC 2010; Smith 2014). Clinical decision making is a day to day activity, one which can involve a high degree of complexity, little time, and a great deal of pressure in which to ensure the right outcome (Smith 2014; Bach and Ellis 2011). Irrespective of these pressures the mental health nurse will always be required to justify the decisions taken and their subsequent actions, sometimes the process of justification may involve looking back at an incident after a great deal of time has elapsed (Smith 2014; NMC 2015a).

To be an effective decision-maker the mental health nurse would need to follow a systematic process which includes (Smith 2014):

- identifying the presenting issue;
- analysing the available evidence;
- considering the options;
- planning the way forward;
- implementing the chosen decision; and
- evaluating the outcome of the decision.

Following a decision-making framework can appear logical and unemotional, however practice decisions, even ones where time is not an issue, will have an emotional context (ibid.). This is why it is vital that the mental health nurse actively engages in critical reflection, by doing so they will have the opportunity to become emotionally intelligent (ibid.). During this reflective process, to increase the accuracy of their decision-making, the mental health nurse should consider the following (Lane and Corrie 2012):

- What is driving your judgement, is it the evidence-base, your intuition or both?
- Be open to the idea that you might be wrong.

- Have you involved all the relevant parties?
- Have you considered different views?

Using the best evidence within the clinical decision-making process is a key part of the clinical decision-making process (Smith 2014). The expectation is that where available the best evidence will be scientific evidence based on current research and following the relevant clinical guidelines, making sense of the evidence includes (ibid.):

- identifying the clinical issue;
- framing the issue as a clinical question;
- searching the available literature;
- critiquing the different forms of evidence;
- delivering the chosen intervention; and
- evaluating the delivery of the chosen intervention.

Systematic approaches to decision-making are useful, however they have to take into account the therapeutic and values-based dimension of mental health nursing (ibid.). Some decisions are straight forward in mental health nursing or so it seems, let us consider John's situation and the 'fact' that he is experiencing delusions. John has been diagnosed with the mental health condition schizophrenia. One of his symptoms is that he experiences delusions; he believes he is doing God's work as his son and that mental health services are conspiring with the Devil to stop him doing this work. This sounds like a delusion; so what is a delusion? Morrison characterises delusion as follows: 'Believing something is true that is not, the individual cannot be persuaded otherwise. These false ideas often involve persecution, such as by government agencies, but others may be grandiose' (Morrison 2014: 186).

This definition is comparable with the seminal work of Jaspers (1913/1997) the core notion being; 'false beliefs'. Defining delusion has been subject to much criticism; therefore delusions are generally understood as false beliefs and that the decision to call a belief a delusion is made by an external observer, usually the psychiatrist (Oyebode 2008). In the case of John a judgement is made by the psychiatrist supported by the mental health team that aspects of John's thinking are delusional. The identified presence of delusional thinking can be seen to be based on the belief that it can be empirically tested and it is not based on a value judgement, in other words it is an objective judgement (Fulford 2009). This judgement, because it is part of the diagnostic process, looks like a fact whereas it is really the case that it is a value, someone makes a judgement that a 'normal person' in society would not hold these beliefs, and as that someone is deemed to be an expert then this value judgement takes on a factual meaning (ibid.).

It is the same in mental health nursing practice where the nurse gathers value judgements that have a factual meaning, beside symptoms this can include clinical risk, what is important is that the nurse is aware that these judgements are value-laden (Roberts 2004; Fulford 2009). To recap, clinical decision-making in mental health nursing practice has to be systematic, however in the real world of practice the nurse has to be aware that facts may be value-based judgement and ones that may have a degree of uncertainty (Lane and Corrie 2012). So, returning to John, let us consider a way forward using a real-world decision-making process (ibid.):

The staff think it would be against John's human rights not to be allowed to sleep when he wants.

- Embrace ambiguity – be aware that things do not always fit into models and systems.
- Work in partnership with the service user and the multi-professional team to solve complex problems.
- Consider all perspectives.

Making decisions which are ethical

When making day-to-day decisions the mental health nurses has to consider that there is uncertainty, facts may be values, and also a service user's freedoms may be restricted (Smith 2012b). These restrictions are usually due to the level of risk the service user poses to themselves and/or others. Where this is the case the mental health nurse is expected to keep the service user safe which is a duty of care (Rylance and Simpson 2012; NMC 2015a). The impact on the mental health nurse decision-making is that the outcomes of those decisions have to be ethical, the nurse has to make a decision which is seen to be right, or has the right motive, or there is a good outcome (Bloch and Green 2009; NMC 2015a).

Making decisions that are ethical requires a great deal of self-awareness especially when in some cases the mental health nurse has the power to control another person by the virtue that they are labelled mentally ill and pose a risk (Horsfield *et al.* 2011; Roberts 2005; Eales 2009). Throughout this use of power the nurse has to maintain a therapeutic relationship that is collaborative even though an increase in risk usually means an increase in the level of control that the mental health nurse exerts over the mental health service user (Roberts 2005; Smith 2012b). To ensure that the mental health nurse is using this power fairly when making decisions there is the expectation that they will reference any relevant ethical and legal frameworks (Smith 2012b; Roberts 2005; Peele and Chodoff 2009). In addition there is the need for the mental health nurse to recognise that mental health nursing practice has a value-laden dimension where ethical conflict can arise if not addressed (Fulford 2009; Chodoff 2009).

By the mental health nurse being critically reflective and understanding the power relationship they have with a mental health service user this increases the chance of reducing ethical conflict (Smith 2012b). Critical reflection can be engendered throughout the therapeutic relationship by using an 'open dialogue' approach; one that is person–centred and respectful of the service user's needs (ibid.).

If we consider the use of the locked door in John's case there may be a good rationale why the door is locked, but what about the emotional impact the locked door is having upon John. By engaging an 'open dialogue' approach the mental health nurse will start to explore this emotional dimension and understand the impact that the locked door is having upon John, something that the nurse may have been unaware of previously (Roberts 2005; Smith 2012b). Truly listening to John's voice will enable the nurse to move beyond labels, it will also give the nurse the opportunity to explore decision-making options with John that may be less restrictive (Roberts 2005; Martinez 2009; Smith 2012b). Ashmore's (2008) study also makes the point that the practice of door locking is at times about mental health services covering their own back by appearing to keep everyone safe rather than being about either good practice or being of benefit to service users.

Ward doors were not always locked on acute mental health wards; the return to door locking can be seen as a return to the practices of the asylum and certainly where door locking is used as a catchall approach which impacts upon all service-users irrelevant of their risk or legal status (Department of Mental Health and Learning Disability 2006; Alexander and Bowers 2004; Ashmore 2008). Locking doors can be seen as the need to be in control, which emanates from the increasing focus over the last decade on containing and minimising risk within mental health services (Ashmore 2008). This focus of containing and minimising risk stems from the social and political perception, or possibly misperception, that mental health service users are risky and possibly more dangerous than the average person in society (Smith 2012b). The subsequent impact upon mental health nursing practice is that politically it is better to lock the door even if does not benefit the service user i.e. to practise defensively than to take a therapeutic risk which in reality may be of more benefit to the service user (Roberts 2005; Ashmore 2008).

The political view holds that door locking will prevent service users engaging in behaviours that can lead to serious harm or death and in turn is an effective way to prevent suicide, even though the vast majority of absconding service users do harm themselves or others, whereas suicides still happen on locked wards (Coppock and Hopton 2000; Ashmore 2008). Locked doors can reduce absconding yet due to the complexity of mental health nursing practice it does not necessarily follow that risk is minimised (Ashmore 2008). Locking doors may actually increase risky behaviours by encouraging service users who cannot leave because the doors are locked to attempt to leave by using more high-risk strategies and by intensifying feelings such as feeling confined, trapped, and frustrated and in turn these feelings could increase both absconding and harming behaviours (ibid.). A report by the Department of Mental Health and Learning Disability found:

> 49 (36%) of the wards were permanently locked, and at the ward level these wards had higher rates of self-harm … Strikingly, many of the other common security practices of acute psychiatry, such as the banning of

harmful items, searches of patient property, and restrictions on patient activities or access to kitchen or bathing facilities appeared to have no association with self-harm rates.

(Department of Mental Health and Learning Disability 2006: 122)

Interestingly where the mental health nurse works with the service user who has a history of absconding to specifically reduce their absconding behaviour, absconding can reduce by as much as 50 per cent (Bowers *et al.* 2003, 2006; Ashmore 2008). Let us return now to the case of John:

> The nurse takes the opportunity to work with John through a process of listening to John's story and reflecting on the lessons that can be learnt (Bowers *et al.* 2003). Listening to John's viewpoint helps the nurse not only to reflect and learn but also to understand the tensions that can arise from door locking (Pang 1999; Bowers *et al.* 2003). Reflecting on John's experiences of a door locking situation gives the nurse an emotional insight into John's experiences and also the opportunity to understand what emotionally does and does not work in that situation (Martinez 2009). Reflecting and listening to John's door locking experiences can be of great value to the mental health nurse in that it will improve their future decision-making in similar incidences and it will also help them address the ethical dimension of their future decision-making.

Key learning points

1 Mental health nurses may not always recognise that the decisions they make have an ethical dimension, in other words this dimension tends to be hidden. To act ethically the mental health nurse has to clinically and ethically reason in a way that is systematic and justifiable.
2 Ethical theories which relate to specifically mental health nursing practice are normative theories which focus on what actions are right, what ought to be done, what motives are good, and what characteristics are virtuous.
3 Mental health nursing in the UK has always been closely aligned with the medical discipline of psychiatry which has largely shaped how mental health nurses practice today.
4 It is important to note that confining and conforming still takes place through the use of implicit and explicit interventions.
5 There is a strong positivist or scientific influence prevalent within contemporary mental health nursing practice. This influence can not only be seen to be prevalent it also can be seen to dominant the way mental health practitioners construct their practice.
6 Mental health nurses also use tacit knowledge which is accrued through the nurse knowing the service user, in other words working with the service user's

story. Mental health nurses should be comfortable working in this way especially nurses who are orientated towards using a talking therapy approach.

7   Mental health nurses are professionally accountable for their practice decisions, they have to be person-centred and partnership focused, they also have to be based on the best available evidence. The process should be systematic with agreed outcomes, and where the nurse does not have the necessary expertise they should signpost appropriately.

8   Clinical decision-making in mental health nursing practice has to be systematic, however in the real world of practice the nurse has to be aware that facts may be value-based judgements and have a degree of uncertainty.

9   When making day-to-day decisions the mental health nurse has to recognise that a service user's freedoms may be restricted. These restrictions are usually due to the level of risk the service user poses to themselves and/or others. Where this is the case the mental health nurse is expected to keep the service user safe which is a duty of care. Using restrictions have to be ethical and they have to be justified.

10 Using restrictions such as a locked door may have a good rationale, however there is still an emotional impact for the service user. By engaging the service user and using an open dialogue approach the mental health nurse will start to work within this emotional dimension and understand the emotional impact that a restriction is having upon the service user. Truly listening to the service user's voice will also enable the nurse to move beyond labels, it will also give the nurse the opportunity to explore decision-making options with the service user that may be less restrictive.

2

THE ETHICAL SELF

Background

The aim of this chapter is to map out the mental health nurse's journey on the way to being an ethical practitioner. This journey is intertwined with the journey towards being an expert practitioner (Smith 2012b). It tends to be viewed as starting at the commencement of the nurse's pre-registration training. Yet in reality it has no boundaries; it starts in early childhood and continues throughout life as part of a person's lifelong learning activities (Smith 2014). It is important to recognise each person's experiences are unique and dynamic, and on this basis their journey towards being an ethical practitioner will also be unique and dynamic (ibid.). During their pre-registration training the student mental health nurse will learn about being ethical, about relevant frameworks. They will also recognise the ethical challenges that can arise during their practice, and, just as important, they will learn about the importance of being self-aware (ibid.; NMC 2010).

Once qualified the mental health nurse is professionally expected to practice ethically while at the same time taking into account the value-laden nature of mental health practice (Smith 2012b; NMC 2015a). To do this the mental health nurse has to be sensitive to the individual context of the care they deliver, being sensitive enables them respond in the right way. It would be easy to say responding in the right way is just about being logical and scientific, however as caring professionals mental health nurses have to also respond at an emotional level, meaning that they have to be emotionally sensitive (Radden 2002; Radden and Sadler 2008). The main way that a mental health nurse can be seen to be emotionally sensitive is through the use of such traits as kindness, patience, tolerance and compassion, to name a few, these traits form an important part of the delivery of the therapeutic relationship, which is the medium of treatment in mental health nursing (Armstrong 2006). It is important to note that though these traits are used throughout all the fields of nursing they also have to be contextualised by the type of nursing. Meaning for the mental health nurse as an example being compassionate within a mental health nursing context is shaped by the nature of mental health nursing which is more coercive than say adult nursing (Roberts 2004; Hursthouse 1999).

Being compassionate is a key part of delivering person-centred care; it is also a trait that nurses as effective communicators should possess (Smith 2014; NMC 2015a; Francis 2013; Commissioning Board 2012). The NMC's (2015a) professional code expects that a nurse will 'treat people with kindness, respect and compassion' (ibid.: 4), and 'when people are in distress the nurse will respond compassionately and kindly' (ibid.: 5). Being an ethical practitioner requires the mental health nurse to be sensitive to the emotional context of a situation, it also requires them to possess 'practical wisdom', the ability to make the right choice when deciding on a course of action, a choice that is right because it is also ethical (Gardiner 2003). A situation which is not handled correctly, expertly and in a sensitive manner may be perceived as abusive practice (Alexander and Bowers 2004; Chodoff 2009). At this juncture let us consider the following scenario which will shape our journey through this chapter:

> Peter has a diagnosis of dementia he is very active and wanders the nursing home day and night. On occasion he becomes aggressive and demands to go home, this type of behaviour happens more often when his wife visits. Due to the lack of staff, constant observation is not possible when Peter wanders and on occasion he has managed to leave the building, he will return quite happily with staff that he finds familiar. At night time there is less staff around to manage Peter's wandering and aggressive behaviour and on this basis he is more likely to be given additional sedation.

Self-awareness

Peter by his actions is telling a story, is anyone truly listening? A key criticism of health and social care services is that they fail to meet service user needs because they do not engage in a way that they truly listen, identify need, and then act upon those identified needs (Alzheimer's Society 2014; Francis 2013). So what is the difference between listening and truly listening? Mental health nursing at times can fall into a way of working that focuses on collecting information and as a consequence true meaning can be lost (Smith 2012a). As an example Peter may be wandering the nursing home because he is bored and has nothing to occupy his time or he may just like to walk, this behaviour that the nurse is observing can become reconstructed into 'Peter wanders which is part of his dementia' (ibid.). It has become a problem to solve in a way that is medicalised, using technical language, and using medical interventions such as medication (ibid.).

In addition using assessment tools and different types of forms can distract the mental health nurse from the need to truly listen (ibid.). Collecting this type of information provides a snapshot of a person in that moment in time, it does not and cannot provide a full picture of the person (Bracken and Thomas 2005). The challenge for the mental health nurse is that listening to the service user's wider story is set against the need to reconstruct and intervene especially where risk is identified, the danger is that this story becomes intellectualised and narrow, a by-product of the assessment process (Smith 2012a; Merleau-Ponty 1945/1962). Listening and being an effective listener and not just intellectualising the service user's narrative requires the nurse to be effective in working with the service user's story, not to interpret the story but to work with the story in the context of the whole person and not take a segmented approach (Hurley and Rankin 2008; Bracken and Thomas 2005).

By looking at only fragments of the client's story the mental health nurse runs the risk of neutralising the story, in effect the meaning of the story is lost (Bracken and Thomas 2005). This happens due to the service user who is the author of the story and who also brings both context and meaning to the story being almost separated from their story. This is a direct result of the mental health nurse placing their own interpretation upon the story, at this point the story is owned by the nurse and ceases to be the service user's story (ibid.; Hamilton and Roper 2006). To prevent this from happening the first thing the mental health nurse has to do is immerse themselves in the story, only thinking about the purpose of the narrative, the content of the messages contained within the narrative, and the overall tone of the narrative and its message (Bracken and Thomas 2005; Shaffer and Zikmund-Fisher 2013).

Sometimes it is difficult to truly listen due to time constraints or not having the right space available. Due to these constraints it is easy to assume certain things about the service user, it also easy to not be aware of any underlying assumptions or values the nurse holds about the service user (Bracken and Thomas 2005). By being self-aware during the listening process this gives the mental health nurse the further opportunity to support the service user in the re-telling of the story, which in itself is a powerful medium for healing (ibid.; Brendel 2006). This process of healing through re-telling is dependent on not only the mental health nurse being empathetic but also on the nurse suspending their intervening attitude during the re-telling process (Wilkin 2006; Hamilton and Roper 2006; Smith 2012a).

Being empathetic is based on being self-aware, being self-aware takes time and is a continuous process, the more self-aware a nurse is the more likely they will be a safe and effective practitioner (Knott 2012). The notion of a self is tricky to pin down, which makes trying to define self-awareness even more difficult. In essence a mental health nurse:

> needs to be aware of the impact their self has upon others, they need to be aware of their own thoughts and feelings, and they also need to be able to use this knowledge in a positive way when working with service users.
>
> (Smith 2014: 5)

To be self-aware the mental health practitioner has to recognise that the self has component parts: the outer component, the self that other people can see and interact with, and the inner component, the self where we have private emotions and thoughts (Knott 2012). To be self-aware the nurse has to be aware of both these components in order to develop and build sustainable therapeutic relationships, (ibid.). The self-aware nurse also has to be skilled in knowing when to disclose this inner world especially as self-disclosure can be a key part of demonstrating empathy (ibid.). Empathy allows the mental health nurse to recognise and acknowledge the emotional world of the service user while still maintaining a sense of their own self (ibid.). Empathic skills include being:

- an active listener;
- genuinely interested;
- accepting the person; and
- caring and compassionate (Smith 2014: 5).

These skills are not things a mental health nurse just does, they have to actively listen and really show interest, it is not just a case of nodding the head at the right time, they also have to be committed to person–centred care moving beyond the service user's diagnostic label (Knott 2012; Shipley 2010). This acceptance of the service user goes back to the mental health nurse needing to immerse themselves within the service user's narrative (Bracken and Thomas 2005; Shaffer and Zikmund-Fisher 2013). Of course the mental health nurse at the same time has to process this information as a professional who has to exercise clinical judgement (NMC 2015a). This is not always easy as mental health nursing can be laden with conflict, and the mental health nurse may believe they are helping the service user whereas the service-user may just view the mental health nurse as an authority figure; someone who has the power to discharge them if they say the right things (Bowers 2010; Smith 2012b). Even when there is conflict the mental health nurse has to do the right thing and act in the correct way and they have to maintain their ethical self (NMC 2015a; Smith 2012b). Returning to Peter:

During the day shift Alex, a newly qualified nurse, is on duty, she notices Peter wandering around and looking a bit tired and grumpy. She asks him what the matter is, and he says he wants to go home. She reassures Peter he is in a nursing home, which is now his home; he is fine with this response and decides to rest for a bit. As the shift proceeds Peter continues to ask Alex every so often when he can go home. After the twentieth occasion Alex becomes frustrated. She then takes a deep breath, reflects, and realises that, due to Peter's memory difficulties, for him this is the first he has asked this question. Alex then responds in the same calm and relaxed manner she did when Peter first asked this question.

Values

Values can be viewed as 'things we value, or are able to find value in' (Duncan 2010: 17). What I may value is not necessarily valued by other people (ibid.). There can be seen three types of values; subjective, instrumental, and intrinsic (ibid.; Dworkin 1995). Subjective values are things we value because we like them or prefer them (Duncan 2010). Instrumental values relate to the usefulness of something and intrinsic value is where something is valued even if it is not useful or necessarily liked (ibid.). As mental health nurses we have personal values, ones that have developed time and which we hold before becoming a nurse (ibid.). We also have professional values that have developed out of becoming a nurse, as an example a nurse should value being person-centred (ibid.). Mental health nurse values will also be influenced by the body of knowledge they work with such as the nature of mental illness and the way they work with their service users through the therapeutic relationship (ibid.; Silverstein 2006).

When working within the therapeutic relationship the mental nurse will work in a way that integrates all their knowledge and skills including the values they hold (Silverstein 2006). As an example the nurse has to be person-centred, they also have to work within an evidence-base that is orientated towards a bio-medical view of mental distress (Chung and Nolan 1994; Silverstein 2006). This bio-medical view is based on the notion that mind body are one and by correcting a neurological abnormality this will also correct a problem pertaining to the individuals psychological functioning (Silverstein 2006; New Scientist 1997). In addition the mental health nurse needs to be person-centred and understand from the mental health service user's perspective or know through the skilled use of empathy their viewpoint (Reynolds 2008; Perraud *et al.* 2006). To do this, which can be a challenge, the mental health nurse has to set aside their own judgements and preconceptions, the bio-medical view, and be attuned to the mental health service user's viewpoint (Reynolds 2008; Perraud *et al.* 2006).

Whatever theory of mental health distress the mental health nurse subscribes to when working within the therapeutic relationship it will have an impact (Chung and Nolan 1994; Silverstein 2006). This impact could shape the very nature of the therapeutic relationship. The mental health nurse who takes a biomedical view may value the therapeutic relationship in a more supportive way, whereas a nurse that takes a more psychosocial view may view the therapeutic relationship as the medium for treatment (Smith 2012a; Silverstein 2006).

As an example 'hearing voices' can be conceptualised as a symptom of mental disorder such as schizophrenia or could be seen as 'someone who hears voices when there is no one around' (Leff 2001; Sims 2003). What matters is the approach; a biomedical approach would intervene primarily using a biological approach such as medication whereas the psychosocial approach would primarily work with the individual's emotional and psychological distress (Leff 2001; Hurley and Rankin 2008). That is not to say that both approaches only use their favoured approach, the psychosocial approach would not necessarily object to the use of medication but it would only be seen as a supportive measure rather than a cure (Bentall 2003).

Mental health nurses are trained to listen and through the therapeutic relationship understand another's experience, however mental health nurses intervene or try to fix things which can result in not listening and in turn not truly understanding the service user's viewpoint and their values (Bertram and Stickley 2005; Wilkin 2006). To manage this conflict the mental health nurse has to be in touch with their feelings and values, they also have to value working in partnership which is underpinned by the commitment to understand and empower (Clarke 2008, 2006; Perraud *et al.* 2006).

To ensure that mental health nurses have the right values they have to act in accordance with the NMC's (2015a) code of conduct. The code cannot help the nurse know how to be ethical in every situation, however it does provide a framework to work within (Smith 2012b). The NMC (2015a) acknowledges that there is always an element of interpretation; 'While you can interpret the values and principles set out in the Code in a range of different practice settings, they are not negotiable or discretionary' (NMC 2015a: 2). In addition, the mental health nurse is expected to uphold the reputation of their profession by trying to 'uphold the standards and values set out in the Code' (ibid.: 15).

This means that the mental health nurse has to ensure their values are aligned with the required professional values which are in essence generic nursing values (NMC 2015a). They also have to contextualise those values within their field of practice paying attention to the role values play at an individual level and at a policy level (Cooper 2009). Of course all parties can have differing values: 'The importance of differences of values in all areas of mental health and social care is widely recognised and has been the basis of a number of national and international policy, training and Service development initiatives' (Mental Health Foundation 2009: 6).

Values and how to manage values also underpin policy documents and training resources these include:

> The recent Chief Nursing Officer's review of mental health nursing in England, *From Values to Action* [DH 2006a], and the Scottish Review of Mental Health Nursing, Rights, Relationships and Recovery [Scottish Executive 2006], both emphasize the important role of values in mental health nursing.
>
> *(Cooper 2009: 25)*

Let us now return to Peter.

There is a conflict of values evident in the scenario. Peter wants to wander, and the staff at night believe this is a problem to be managed. The staff have chosen to use medication. They could have chosen not to use medication and see if Peter's rest–wake cycle can be managed in a different way.

Therapeutic relationships

In this section we will tease out the ethical nature of the therapeutic relationship. If we consider the chapter scenario the mental health nurse is starting to build a therapeutic relationship with Peter this should also extend to his family (Smith 2014). This process is built on the mental health nurse using both an evidence-base and paying attention to theirs and others values, this includes recognising Peter needs to be kept safe, however to do this there may be some difficult emotional decisions to be made along the way (Roberts 2004; Smith 2014). Some of these difficult emotional decisions will also have an ethical dimension such as respecting Peter's autonomy, being person-centred, and also keeping Peter safe which may include restricting certain freedoms (Roberts 2004; Bloch and Green 2006). In these types of situations the mental health nurse needs has to be emotionally responsive to how Peter and his family feel about a proposed course of action but also to recognising Peter's vulnerability in that Peter, due to his mental state, may find it difficult to make a reasoned decision (Roberts 2004).

The mental health nurse is the treater and the effectiveness of the therapeutic relationship is dependent on the character of the treater (Radden 2002). So in reference to the scenario the mental health nurse being able to effectively reason and emotionally respond appropriately is dependent on their character and their ability to use such character traits as being trust-worthy, motivated, and empathic (Roberts 2004; NMC 2015a). It is important to note that though character and its corresponding traits are important equally important is the application of those character traits (Radden and Sadler 2008; NMC 2015a). As an example, being empathetic to Peter and his family is important but it is also key when doing the right thing that the mental health nurse knows what communication skills to use and when (Armstrong et al. 2000; Welsh and Lyons 2001).

Knowing the right thing to do or to discern well is based on a number of factors first of all the mental health practitioner needs to possess the correct character traits and values, but also they need to be skilled in their application (McKie and Swinton 2000; Smith and Godfrey 2002; NMC 2015a). This process of possessing and also being skilled in the right character traits and values comes from the mental health nurse's training, and their subsequent practice experiences (Radden and Sadler 2008; Welsh and Lyons 2001). Knowing how to do the right thing is also based on the mental health nurse assessing the situation and then deciding the right course of action. The subsequent interventions the nurse then delivers will only be effective where they have a robust relationship with Peter and his family (Radden 2002). This includes managing risk, the therapeutic relationship is intended to be collaborative and person-centred this intention is dependent on risk, so where Peter's behaviour is deemed to be 'low risk' then the approach can be more collaborative but this becomes more difficult in the case of working with high risk behaviours such as aggression towards others (Perraud et al. 2006; Wilkin 2006; Roberts 2005). At this higher level of risk the therapeutic relationship becomes more controlling and confining until the level of risk is again deemed to be low (Roberts 2005; Smith 2012b).

In relation to Peter the mental health nurse is being empathetic to Peter's situation and will be focused on achieving a collaborative solution to his situation (Perraud *et al.* 2006; Wilkin 2006). Even though Peter is deemed to have a mental health condition in this case dementia, have diminished judgement and be a potential risk to others, the mental health nurse would still be empathetic and collaborative but they would also be looking to control any perceived risk (Smith 2012b; Roberts 2005; Bloch and Green 2006).

To manage risk within the therapeutic relationship the mental nurse will use their discretion; a newly qualified nurse may refer more often to the rules when using discretion whereas the discretion of the expert mental health nurse will not rely solely on the rules (Benner 1982). The use of discretion in this way is shaped by their reflections upon their practice experiences which assist the mental health nurse to deal effectively with the most complex situations (Welsh and Lyons 2001; Alexander and Bowers 2004). Expertly knowing within a mental health nursing context is developed through experience or knowing by doing, this can accrue by observing expert role models demonstrating this and also by reflecting, in turn learning from those reflections (Welsh and Lyons 2001; Schön 1983). While using discretion the mental health nurse has to go with the flow, an Taoist notion, which has to be uncomplicated and simple; it must have a natural and a sensitive rhythm (Hoff 1994; Inada 1995). Gardiner (2003) from a western virtue ethics perspective calls this possessing practical wisdom; the ability to make virtuous choices through learning to use reasoning that is also sensitive to the emotional context of a situation. Returning to going with the flow according to Cheng-tek Tai (2004: 3) adjusting to the flow is a process of 'action without artificiality and arbitrariness' where overacting can become more 'harmful than good'. In other words a mental health nurse going with the flow must avoid making things happen; Cheng-tek Tai (2004: 3) provides a 'symbolic' example of how this approach works in action:

> here is someone who is naturally violent … what shall I do? Be on guard, be careful and be sure that you yourself are acting appropriately. Appear to be flexible but maintain harmony within … While being flexible, be sure to remain centered.
>
> *(Cheng-tek Tai 2004: 5)*

Flexibility is key in going with the flow, but this needs to be tempered by 'centring', as highlighted by Cheng-tek Tai (2004: 5): 'acting has to be natural and spontaneous' but also 'the wise at the same time remain impartial'. A study by Hansson *et al.* (2007: 6) articulates that in stressful doctor-patient situations doctors who act in a genuine manner are more likely to be seen as acting ethically. Obviously acting genuinely has to be real, also it should convey through non-verbal behaviour a sense of genuineness which can also be seen to be natural and spontaneous (Hansson *et al.* 2007; Cheng-tek Tai 2004). Let us return to the chapter scenario to consider how this would work in action.

> When working with Peter the nurse recognises that to be more expert they need to reflect on their work with Peter in a way that is structured. They also recognise that by being an effective communicator they will be able to deliver a range of appropriate psychological interventions such as cognitive stimulation and cognitive rehabilitation focused activities (Smith 2014). As Peter's verbal communication has been severely disrupted the nurse starts to consider Peter's non-verbal communication which includes considering why he wanders. Speaking to Peter's family the nurse realises that Peter is a keen gardener. On this basis the nurse works out a way that Peter can safely access a small courtyard garden. Over a period of time it is noted that, since being able to access the garden, Peter is sleeping at night and wandering less, and there has been a significant reduction in the use of sedating medication.

Effective communication

On qualifying it is expected that the newly qualified mental health nurse will:

- have excellent communication, interpersonal and therapeutic skills;
- be skilled in working in partnership with service users and carers;
- engage in person–centred care which is compassionate and empowering; and
- preserve dignity, be anti-discriminatory, and practise within the law (Smith 2014: 3).

At post-qualification the mental health nurse professionally has to practise effectively and they must communicate clearly. In addition:

- use terms that people in your care, colleagues and the public can understand;
- take reasonable steps to meet people's language and communication needs, providing, wherever possible, assistance to those who need help to communicate their own or other people's needs;
- use a range of verbal and non-verbal communication methods, and consider cultural sensitivities, to better understand and respond to people's personal and health needs;
- check people's understanding from time to time to keep misunderstanding or mistakes to a minimum;
- be able to communicate clearly and effectively in English; and
- use all forms of spoken, written and digital communication (including social media and networking sites) responsibly, respecting the right to privacy of others at all times (NMC 2015a: 7–8, 16).

So when communicating the mental health nurse has to ensure that their communication is framed by the values of their profession with the assumption that if it does it will be effective (Smith 2014). Having effective communication skill will form a solid platform for the mental health nurse to build positive therapeutic relationships and to deliver a broad range of psychological interventions (Knott 2012). In addition the mental health nurse has to manage the tension between being person-centred and empowering and needing to managing risk. This does not mean that risk management is all about control, it can and should be enabling (DH 2010). Returning to Peter's situation rather than looking at Peter's wandering as behaviour to be controlled the nurse should consider it as a form of communication, they have to recognise the risk element, however rather than trying to stop the behaviour they should try and direct it into more positive and enabling activities, hence the gardening activity (ibid.). Risk enablement is framed by the following four steps (ibid.):

1   Understand the person's needs.
2   Understand the impact of risks on the person.
3   Enable and manage risk.
4   Devise a risk plan.

In addition:

> A good risk assessment should demonstrate that risk has been assessed and managed taking into account all perspectives and all aspects of the individual's needs. Practitioners should demonstrate that they have used all means available to skilfully communicate with the person with dementia to best understand their individual needs and wishes.
>
> *(DH 2010: 44)*

We again arrive back at the effective use of communication skills with the emphasis on the mental health nurse to skilfully facilitate what should be a two-way process where information is seamlessly exchanged between the nurse and the service user (Knott 2012). Of course this process can be disrupted especially where a service user is struggling to make sense of shared reality or they have difficulty in expressing themselves verbally, nevertheless the responsibility to get this process back on track lies with the mental health nurse (Smith 2014; NMC 2015a). This requires the nurse to understand what the issue is and then devise a strategy to overcome any difficulties (Smith 2014). Peter was mainly communicating through the use of his non-verbal communication, the nurse recognised this. Most of our communication is non-verbal though there is a tendency to be dependent on focusing on the way a person communicates verbally. Where verbal communication is disputed this type of communication is not a luxury the nurse can rely on; they have to go back to basics and focus on a person's non-verbal communication (Smith 2014; Knott 2012):

- Facial expressions, do they look happy, sad, etc.
- Does the service user maintain eye contact? If not what are they looking at?
- What gestures do they use?
- What posture are they in at the time of communicating?
- How are they using head movements
- Are they using personal space appropriately?
- What does their appearance look like, are they unkempt?

As the communication process is a two-way process the mental health nurse has to be aware of the way they are communicating non-verbally, what is the potential impact their non-verbal communication will have on the service user (Kott 2012). In their response which will effectively be a psychological intervention the mental health nurse will need to acknowledge that the service user could be vulnerable and that the care they deliver has to be compassionate (Smith 2014; NMC 2015a). Compassionate communication has to also be part of a set of baseline communication skills, values, and behaviours called the 6Cs (Smith 2014; Commissioning Board 2012). Returning to the scenario, let us consider these in action:

- *Care* – The nurse should deliver care to Peter that has been tailored to meet his specific needs.
- *Compassion* – The nurse should be intelligently kind towards Peter.
- *Competence* – The nurse should have the expertise to deliver the right care at the right time.
- *Communication* – The nurse's communication should be effective and inclusive.
- *Courage* – The nurse has do the right thing which includes being Peter's advocate.
- *Commitment* – The nurse should place Peter at the centre of the therapeutic relationship.

Key learning points

1 Being an expert mental health nurse and being an ethical mental health nurse are part of the same journey. This lifelong learning journey in reality has no boundaries and continues throughout a person's life. Each nurse's journey is unique and dynamic and to understand the lessons they learn on this journey the nurse has to be self-aware.
2 Being compassionate is a professional trait that nurses as effective communicators should possess.
3 Being an ethical practitioner requires the mental health nurse to possess practical wisdom which is the ability to make the right choice at the right time.
4 The challenge for the mental health nurse is that listening to the service user's wider story is set against the need to reconstruct and intervene. Truly listening

and not just intellectualising the service user's narrative requires the nurse to be effective in working with the service user's story in a holistic way.

5   What I may value is not necessarily valued by other people (Duncan 2010). There are three types of value; subjective, instrumental and intrinsic. As mental health nurses we have personal values ones that have developed usually before becoming a nurse and professional values that develop out of becoming a nurse.

6   Mental health nurses' values will also be influenced by the body of knowledge they work with, such as the nature of mental illness, and this impacts on the way they work therapeutically with service users.

7   The mental health nurse needs to be emotionally responsive at all times, recognising a service user's vulnerability and how difficult it may be to make a reasoned decision.

8   The mental health nurse is the treater and the effectiveness of the therapeutic relationship is dependent on the character of the treater. The mental health nurse being able to effectively reason and emotionally respond is dependent on their character and their ability to use such character traits as being trustworthy, motivated and empathic.

9   When communicating the mental health nurse has to ensure that their communication is framed by the values of their profession with the assumption that if it does it will be effective.

10   The mental health nurse has to manage the tension between being person-centred and empowering and the need to manage risk. This does not mean that risk management is all about control, it can and should be enabling.

3

ETHICAL REASONING

A pragmatic approach

Background

The aim of this chapter is to introduce ethical reasoning as a systematic and balanced process that mental health nurses can use in their day-to-day practice. Each component of this process will be explored in more detail in the rest of this book.

Cleary *et al.* (2012) describes mental health nursing practice within acute settings as fast paced where mental health nurses have to deal with difficult circumstances. Commonly the nurse's response to these conditions is to interact with service users in a way that is fluid, non-confrontational, and pragmatic; their response is shaped by the situation they are dealing with (Cleary *et al.* 2012; Bowers *et al.* 2009). During this process the mental health nurse has to make the right decisions, they have to ethically reason and in a way that they can justify their decisions (Cohen 2004; NMC 2015a). To assist in making ethically justifiable decisions the mental health nurse is expected to follow a professional code of conduct in this case the NMC's (2015a) code of conduct (Coady 2009). This code is there to assist the nurse to make a decision, it is also there 'to protect the public. We do this by making sure that only those who meet our requirements are allowed to practise as a nurse or midwife in the UK. We take action if concerns are raised about whether a nurse or midwife is fit to practise' (NMC 2015a: 19).

Ethical theories also have a role to play in having a direct influence on the ethical decision-making process (Cohen 2004). This role is not always evident to mental health nurses and yet nurses will, when reflecting on clinical situations, talk about an action that is right or wrong, or they will talk about having a bad or good attitude, which relate directly to a number of ethical theories (Smith 2012b; Bloch and Green 2009). These theories which we discuss in more detail later in the book have a top-down influence in that they can provide a framework or set of principles that a mental health nurse can use to frame their justification (Cohen 2004). Codes of conduct are also influenced by ethical theories using terms such as values, duties, rights, among other terms (Ford 2006). Mental health nurses in addition to top-down reasoning will engage in bottom-up reasoning (Cohen 2004). This is where a practice situation will generate what Cohen (ibid.: 61) calls a 'moral reaction', a situation that needs to be reasoned through, these occur on a daily basis and are an integral part of clinical decision-making. On this basis mental health nurses will be pre-dominantly bottom-up ethical reasoners, to take a balanced approach they will also have to engage in top-down reasoning at the same time (ibid.; NMC 2015a).

Let us consider the following chapter scenario.

Sally is a second-year pre-registration mental health nursing student who has been on an acute mental health ward for the last six weeks. Sally has enjoyed her placement; she feels as if this is her first real mental health placement. The ward is busy and there is lots of activity. She notices that most of the time her mentor is in the office doing paperwork. Yet to Sally's surprise her mentor appears to have good relationship with the service users and appears to know what is going on at all times. Another mystery is that when dealing with complex situations her mentor does the right thing, but cannot always articulate immediately after the situation how they worked through it. However, a couple of days later they then have a good rational explanation.

Moral development

Being able to ethically reason is an activity that is connected with a person's development; this starts in early childhood (Gross 2015). Psychological theories of moral development are influenced by the work of Piaget and Kohlberg. This work encompasses a person's moral or ethical development from the early stages of childhood to adulthood and in reference to society's moral rules (ibid.). Other theorists have studied moral development; however, this section will focus on the work of Piaget and Kohlberg. Piaget took the view that at first a child's ethical reasoning was heavily influenced by authority figures, however over time they became more independent and used ethical rules to make sense of their reasoning (ibid.). Kohlberg built upon Piaget's work and developed a staged approach to moral development (ibid.). In essence Kohlberg's approach has six stages which are grouped into three levels and correspond to age. As the child passes through each stage on the way to adulthood their ethical reasoning becomes more effective (ibid.). These stages as a summary include:

1   Pre-conventional
    –   Obedience and punishment orientation
    –   Self-interest orientation
2   Conventional
3   Interpersonal accord and conformity

4   Authority and social-order maintaining orientation
5   Social contract orientation
6   Universal ethical principles (Gross 2015).

Children will ethically reason at the pre-conventional stage and adults at the conventional stage and beyond (ibid.). An initial feature of the conventional stage is that a person follows society's rules and this shapes their sense of what is right and what is wrong (ibid.). Over time their behaviour starts to correspond to what right and wrong look like, it is viewed as good to be seen as a good person, feedback from others starts to influence this process, and it is good to be seen as a good person. The person recognises that to effectively function within a wider social context it is important to follow society's rules. Most people can be seen to operate at this stage however Kohlberg added two extra stages which include being able to ethically reason in an abstract way (ibid.). The individual starts to recognise that everyone holds different opinions and views and should be respected, and in addition will challenge these views if they do not agree (Baxter and Boblin 2007). Gilligan (1982), in response to Kohlberg's theory, developed a model that took into account the female view; 'She suggested that women have a distinct moral voice and describe moral situations using a distinct language' (Baxter and Boblin 2007: 22).

Gilligan's model has three perspectives (ibid.):

• Caring for the self to ensure survival.
• A maternal morality that seeks to ensure care for the dependent and unequal.
• A focus on the dynamics of relationships and the resolution of tension between selfishness and responsibility for others.

Rest (1986) developed a four-component model, with morality dependent on how an individual cognitively interacts with a situation (Baxter and Boblin 2007):

1   Interpretation of the situation.
2   Decision regarding a course of action.
3   Conflict of other values with moral values.
4   Execution and implementation of a plan of action.

The implication for nursing is:

> Nurses are guided in their everyday lives by their personal values and beliefs about what is right and good. Such personal beliefs define nurses' sense of morality and influence how they customarily make decisions and react to usual problems .
>
> *(Cohen and Erickson 2006: 776, citing Fletcher, Miller and Spencer 1997)*

Nurses have to deal with complex and difficult situations where their own ethical development will come into play (Cohen and Erickson 2006). In addition their pre-registration training and their post-qualifying experiences will further shape this development (ibid.). On this basis it is suggested that 'Kohlberg's theory, however, needs to be adjusted in relation to nursing care … The abstract, rigid and justice-oriented ethical concept seems to be inadequate for nursing practice' (Dierckx de Casterlé *et al.* 2008: 542, citing Dierckx de Casterlé *et al.* 1998).

It is suggested that nurses ethically reason at a post-conventional level where rules provide a framework in addition to the nurse's ability to critically reflect, a higher cognitive skill (Dierckx de Casterlé *et al.* 2008). This ability to critical reflect in the moment is not an unusual feature of expert clinical practice, from an outside perspective this is seen as the expert acting in the right way even in the most difficult situations where accurate information may not be available (Berg 2008; Welsh and Lyons 2001). The expert nurse responds correctly because their experience through the process of critical reflection has become knowledge and they now intuitively know what to do in a difficult clinical situation (Welsh and Lyons 2001; Hardy *et al.* 2002). That is not to say that rules do not have a part to play however, rules can sometimes send the nurse in the wrong direction such as the inexperienced nurse who sticks to the rules and struggles to make sense of a fast moving situation which is new to them (Alexander and Bowers 2004). Whereas the experienced nurse works with the rules and using their experience feels for the right answer as the situation evolves through constant reflection (Welsh and Lyons 2001). In essence expertise becomes a character trait of the expert nurse allowing them to ethically reason at a pre-conventional level (Berg 2008; Dierckx de Casterlé *et al.* 2008). We will now return to Sally.

> Sally asks her mentor about this aspect of knowing the right thing to do. The mentor explains that they always think about their practice in real-time and after an event, they actively engage in clinical supervision which provides a structure to the way they reflect on their practice, and they constantly seek others opinions with a focus on engaging within a critical conversation.

Professional expectations

During the care they deliver, mental health nurses work within and implement rules and strategies on a daily basis, sometimes these rules and strategies need to be controlling (Alexander and Bowers 2004; Roberts 2005). Manging and controlling clinical risk, preventing harm to self and others, is a big part of the mental health nurse role, the challenge for the nurse is to ensure they effectively manage risk while at the same time making sure that their therapeutic relationships are enabling and recovery-focused (Department of Mental Health and Learning Disability 2006; Smith 2014). To take a balanced approach and manage clinical risk while being recovery-focused, the mental health nurse will have to constantly reflect on their practice (NMC 2015a). This requires an ability to reason at a high level and also appreciate that clinical reasoning is not a separate exercise to ethical reasoning, they are one and the same process (Smith 2012b; Dierckx de Casterlé *et al.* 2008). During this process the nurse will have to frame their reasoning through the relevant rules which includes acknowledging the professional expectation that they will do the right thing (Smith 2012b; Mitchell 2011). Professionally for the mental health nurse, doing the right thing is located within NMC's (2015a) code of conduct, this code is there to ensure that the public are protected and any practice that is not in accordance with the code may lead to various professional sanctions (Coady 2009; NMC 2015a). As an overview, 'The Code contains a series of statements that taken together signify what good nursing and midwifery practice looks like. It puts the interests of patients and service users first, is safe and effective, and promotes trust through professionalism' (NMC 2015a: 3).

These statements provide structure to the code as main headings:

- prioritise people;
- practise effectively;
- preserve safety; and
- promote professionalism and trust.

Under each main heading further detail is provided through a detailed overview of what the main heading means professionally and then through a number of sub-statements which highlight what a nurse should or should not do. As an example under the main heading 'prioritise people':

> You put the interests of people using or needing nursing or midwifery services first. You make their care and safety your main concern and make sure that their dignity is preserved and their needs are recognised, assessed and responded to. You make sure that those receiving care are treated with respect, that their rights are upheld and that any discriminatory attitudes and behaviours towards those receiving care are challenged.
>
> *(NMC 2015a: 4)*

And the five following sub-statements:

1 Treat people as individuals and uphold their dignity.
2 Listen to people and respond to their preferences and concerns.
3 Make sure that people's physical, social and psychological needs are assessed and responded to.
4 Act in the best interests of people at all times.
5 Respect people's right to privacy and confidentiality.

This pattern continues throughout the code; practising effectively emphasises the need to be responsive, utilise best practice, be an effective communicator, and reflect in a way that leads to action (NMC 2015a). The sub-statements include:

- Always practise in line with the best available evidence.
- Communicate clearly.
- Work cooperatively.
- Share your skills, knowledge and experience for the benefit of people receiving care.
- Keep clear and accurate records relevant to your practice.
- Be accountable for your decisions to delegate tasks and duties to other people.

Preserving safety focuses on ensuring the service user is safe, that the nurse knows their limits, and they concerns (NMC 2015a). The sub-statements include:

- Recognise and work within the limits of your competence.
- Be open and candid with all service users about all aspects of care and treatment.
- Always offer help if an emergency arises in your practice setting or anywhere else.
- Act without delay if you believe that there is a risk to patient safety or public protection.
- Raise concerns immediately if you believe a person is vulnerable or at risk.
- Advise on, prescribe, supply, dispense or administer medicines within the limits of your training and competence, the law, our guidance and other relevant policies, guidance and regulations.
- Be aware of, and reduce as far as possible, any potential for harm associated with your practice.

Promoting professionalism and trust is concerned with ensuring the nurse is committed to upholding the values of the code both in their work life and personal life, and they display these values as a leader and as a role model (NMC 2015a). The sub-statements include:

- Uphold the reputation of your profession at all times.
- Uphold your position as a registered nurse or midwife.
- Fulfil all registration requirements.
- Cooperate with all investigations and audits.
- Respond to any complaints made against you professionally.
- Provide leadership to make sure people's wellbeing is protected.

Let us now return to Sally.

Sally has been reading the code, and one statement Sally resonates with is 'act in the best interests of people at all times'. While reflecting on this statement, Sally thinks about incidences where service users have been admitted to hospital against their will. They do not want to be in hospital and they do not want to receive treatment; however, through a legal process they have been admitted to hospital and have received treatment. Some of these service users in retrospect agree with this decision, others do not. Sally feels confused by this state of affairs and is now not sure what this statement means in practice, especially who determines what is in the best interest of a person.

Rules and their limits

The NMC's code of conduct provides guidelines on how the nurse should practice, however these are general guidelines which require a level of interpretation on the part of the nurse (Smith 2012b; NMC 2015a). For example 'acting in the best interests of people at all times' it is a general statement, the nurse knows that they must do this, it is up to them to decide how, and if required provide a reasonable level of justification for the actions they subsequently undertook (Smith 2012b; NMC 2015a). The law works in a similar way if we look at the Mental Capacity Act (MCA) 2005:

> The MCA applies to situations where you may be unable to make a particular decision at a particular time, to the extent that you cannot do one or more of the points above. For example, someone with dementia may be unable to retain information long enough to make decisions. Or someone with a mental health problem may feel too depressed to make a decision that he or she is able to make when feeling less depressed. In both these instances it may be the case that the person lacks the capacity to make particular decisions at particular times.
>
> *(Mental Capacity Implementation Programme 2009: 8–9)*

Assessing mental capacity requires the practitioner to consider that:

> The Act makes use of a 'functional' test of capacity, adapted from the common law, which focuses on the decision-making process itself. First it must be established that the person being assessed has 'an impairment of, or a disturbance in the functioning of, the mind or brain' which may affect their ability to make the decision in question. Under the Act, a person is regarded as being unable to make a decision if, at the time the decision needs to be made, he or she is unable:

- to understand the information relevant to the decision
- to retain the information relevant to the decision
- to use or weigh the information; or
- to communicate the decision (by any means).

Where an individual fails one or more parts of this test, then they do not have the relevant capacity and the entire test is failed.

(British Medical Association 2008: 10–11)

How does the practitioner know whether someone 'understands the information relevant to the decision'? The starting place is to enter into a dialogue with the person and elicit their understanding or gather 'the facts', the practitioner then has to make a decision based on the information they have gathered and use their professional judgement to decide whether a person understands the information relevant to the decision (Bloch and Green 2006). The key issue of determining whether a person has capacity following this process appears to be fairly straight-forward; it is something that can be established as a fact, if a person does not have capacity, just by following a rational and reasoned process (Beauchamp and Childress 2009). In reality accumulating facts which are really values is a way of supporting and justifying what is really a value-laden judgement, a moral decision rather than a scientific one (Roberts 2004; Fulford 2009).

Again like the code of conduct the law can only provide a framework in which the nurse must rely on their own ability to ethically reason (Smith 2012b; Ford 2006). To be an effective ethical reasoner the nurse has to be able to identify the ethical issues which means they have to be morally sensitive, this skill is accrued through the nurse actively engaging with critical reflection as a structured process (Fulford et al. 2006; Smith 2012b; Comrie 2012). Ethical sensitivity has a number of definitions; in essence it is about the ability to be responsive to the ethical dimension of a service user's situation and to respond accordingly (Comrie 2012). Ethical sensitivity is different depending on the level of experience the nurse has; the more junior the member of staff, the more they look for rules, have they been broken, have they not? More experienced nurses will also look at the ethical values inherent within the therapeutic relationship (ibid.). In addition, working in differ-ent environments can present different ethical dilemmas. For example working on in-patient mental health wards can be difficult environments to work within with acknowledged difficulties highlighted by Currid (2009: 40–41) such as 'poor patient safety, risk of physical and sexual abuse, few opportunities for therapeutic activities, high staff vacancy rates, bed shortages and crisis-driven care'. On this basis the complex, intensive, and restrictive nature of mental health nursing practice within acute mental health means that it is not always clear how the mental health nurse should morally act in situations that can be interpreted in different ways (Bolmsjo et al. 2006; Barker 2011).

Restricting or controlling an individual's freedoms is an issue that has been widely debated by political and legal philosophers interested in coercion (Anderson 2008). At a societal level coercion generally can be seen as a way of 'getting others to do or not do something' with the implication that coercion diminishes the other person's freedom and responsibility, and that it is a wrong and/or violation of rights (Anderson 2008; Carr 1988). On this basis coercion is justified where it is authorised by society such as in the case of preventing the harming of others or the further harming of others (Anderson 2008). Ripstein (2004) views authorised coercion as necessary and justified; 'both the use of official force and the claim of states to tell people what to do are justified because, in their absence, arbitrary individual force prevails, even if people act in good faith' (ibid.: 3). The implication of this view within mental health nursing is that where coercive measures are sanctioned by the 'state' then they can be seen as justified, however if they are not sanctioned then they are not justified (Ripstein 2004). Within a mental health nursing context, O'Brien and Golding (2003) defined coercion as 'any use of (sanctioned) authority by the mental health nurse to override the choices of the respective mental health service user' (ibid.: 168–169).

Coercion in this context can be easily identified in the overt use of restraint, but it can also be more difficult to identify where restraint is not used in the case of the service user who is pressured into taking medication (Smith 2012b; Verkerk *et al.* 2008). At this point we return to the chapter scenario.

Sally is on duty one day when a service user is being admitted on section 3 of the Mental Health Act. The service user is angry and does not want to be in hospital. The service user is known to the ward, none of the staff that know the service user are on duty. The service user on entry to the ward starts to pace and also shouts that they want to go home. The nurse in charge after consulting with the admitting doctor decides to offer the service user oral medication. The service user declines and starts to become verbally abusive. The service user runs towards the ward doors, realises the doors are locked, grabs a member of staff and demands they let them out. The member of staff refuses and is subsequently hit. Almost immediately the service user is restrained, alarms start going off and staff run to the incident. After a few minutes the service user is given an injection and they agree to go into a side-room. Sally feels quite upset when she goes home.

A systematic and balanced approach to ethical reasoning

There are a number of factors that need to be taken into account during the ethical decision-making process. This section will summarise some of these factors ending with an overview of a structured ethical decision-making process. The stages of this process will then be systematically explored throughout the rest of this book. This model will only provide a method in which to systematically work through an ethical problem, identifying the problem is something only the nurse can do and they may have their own individual view of what the problem is (Smith 2012b; Ford 2006). For example a mental health service user is not adhering to their medication regime and repeatedly becomes unwell, which includes a level of risk that necessitates admission to in-patient services. The psychiatrist's view might be that to stay well the service user ought to take their medication; the service user's view is they feel physically unwell when they take their medication, so why should they take it? The nurse's view is that the service user is not engaging with them and they keep stopping taking their medication, by not engaging it reduces the opportunity to explore other options.

This ambiguity creates ethical conflict and on this basis any an ethical reasoning process has to be able to support this nurse in effectively manging this conflict (Smith 2012b; Ford 2006). Another issue to consider is time, situations may well relate to a high level of risk, however the nurse may have the time to systematically work through the issue. This is not always the case, the nurse may well have to act quickly and that is why it is stressed throughout this chapter that the nurse has to, through critical reflection, develop post-conventional ethical reasoning skills (Dierckx de Casterlé *et al.* 2008). A study by Morrison and Symes (2011) found that:

> Common characteristics, grounded in emotional involvement, of expert nursing practice revealed in this review were knowing the patient, intuitive knowledge, reflective practice, risk taking, and skilled know-how, which were demonstrated across many and varied nursing specialty settings.
>
> *(Morrison and Symes 2011: 169)*

An important point to note is being expert cannot happen in isolation there has to be an organisational commitment to support the nurse towards being an expert. Expert practice will be looked at in more detail later in the book. It is also important to recognise that there are a number of ethical reasoning processes available, some are more generic than others. For example Rhodes and Alfandre (2007) offer a model which is principle-based and quite time consuming, however it does focus on guiding a person to resolve the issue at hand:

- collect all the information relevant to the issue;
- identify principles involved;
- consider whether these principles conflict;
- decide which principle should have priority;
- when uncertainty persists is there missing information that would help;
- evaluate your decision; and
- action plan.

The reason this model is time consuming is that there is a constant need to keep looking for information to help the nurse decide which principle they should be using, which is derived from the ethical theory of principlism. We will look at principlism later in the book.

The ethical reasoning process used in this book is similar to the Rhodes and Alfandre (2007) process, however it does not locate itself in one particular ethical theory. In addition it will not resolve the time-consuming issue completely but it is adaptive enough to fit within the nurse's reflective endeavours (Smith 2012b; Ford 2006; Bolmsjo *et al.* 2006). The following is an overview of the model:

1   Recognise the ethical issue/s.
2   Gather the facts and values.
3   Consider the rules.
4   Look at any underpinning moral theories.
5   Consider all options.
6   Make a decision and test it.
7   Act and reflect on the outcome.

As mental health practice based on risk can restrict certain freedoms there is a need to factor this into the process (Roberts 2004; Smith 2012b). An appropriate place based on the work of Woodbridge and Fulford (2004) would be at the facts and values stage – 'two feet principle'. This approach provides a practice approach to resolving ethical conflict within mental health practice and one that is recovery-focused (Cleary *et al.* 2013). Mental health nurses are constantly balancing the need to manage risk which potentially restricts freedoms, and being collaborative, respecting the autonomy of person (Roberts 2005; Smith 2012b). The more restrictive the nurse has to be the more likely ethical issues will arise, not all these issues are identified due to the value-laden nature of mental health practice (Goethals *et al.* 2013). The nurse may focus on managing risk believing they are acting in the best interests of the service user, they will probably have lots of evidence to justify their actions, however the service user despite the nurse's justification believes that their freedoms are being unjustly restricted (Smith 2012b). Listening to the service user and identifying the values inherent within the situation provides a starting place towards manging this conflict and in addition potentially resolving this conflict (Goethals *et al.* 2013).

The mental health nurse must also recognise that they come from a position of power; they have power to monitor and the power to intervene or control (Roberts 2005). This power is sanctioned by society and can take the form of explicit power, rules and regulations, and implicit power mental health nursing interventions which are based on managing risk (ibid.). Recognising the power they hold within the therapeutic relationship puts the emphasis on the mental health nurse to be committed to actively take into account the service users viewpoint and their subsequent values, the core of their practice (Lamza and Smith 2014). Skilfully paying attention to the service user's values requires the mental health nurse to do the following:

1   Consider the service user's perspective
2   It is important to consider codes of conduct and moral theories, but are these approaches balanced, have you considered the service user's values and narrative?
3   Make sure that the service user's story does not lose its person-centred element.
4   Listen to the service user's account and make sure that this account is fully represented.

When Sally is next on duty she talks to her mentor about the incident and works through some of her concerns. Sally decides to have a chat with the service user to explore their view of the incident. The service user says to Sally, 'I was angry. How would you feel being locked when you have done nothing wrong?'

Key learning points

1   Mental health nursing practice can be complex and fast paced where mental health nurses have to deal with difficult circumstances. The nurse's response to these conditions is shaped more by the situation than a set of rigid rules. During this process the mental health nurse has to make the right decision and they have to justify that decision.

2   Mental health nurses are expected to follow a professional code of conduct in this case the NMC's (2015a) code of conduct which is there to assist the nurse in making the right decision.

3   Being able to ethically reason is an activity that is heavily connected with a person's psycho-social development. There are a number of psychological theories of moral development which have been heavily influenced by the work of Piaget and Kohlberg.

4   Kohlberg built upon Piaget's work and developed a staged approach to moral development. In essence ethical reasoning has six stages which are grouped into three levels and correspond to age.

5   Mental health nurses work within and implement rules and strategies on a daily basis, there is also the element of needing to control the clinical situation and manage clinical risk.

6   To take a balanced approach, manging clinical risk and being recovery-focused, the mental health nurse will need to constantly think about their practice which requires an ability to reason at a high level and also appreciate that clinical reasoning is not a separate exercise to ethical reasoning, they are one and the same process.

7   During this process the nurse will have to frame their reasoning through the relevant rules which includes acknowledging the professional expectation that they will do the right thing. The code is used to ensure that the public are protected and any practice that is not in accordance with the code may lead to various professional sanctions.

8   The NMC's code of conduct provides guidelines on how the nurse should act, however these are general guidelines which require a level of interpretation on the part of the nurse, the law works in a similar way.

9   There are a number of factors that need to be taken into account during the ethical decision–making process. Any model will only provide a method in which to systematically work through an ethical problem, identifying the

problem is something only the nurse can do and they may have their own individual view of what the problem is.

10 Ambiguity can create ethical conflict, on this basis any ethical reasoning process has to be able to support the nurse in effectively manging this conflict. Another issue to consider is time, situations may well relate to a high level of risk, however the nurse may not have lots of time to systematically work through the issue, they may need to work through a situation at that moment in time.

4

RECOGNISING ETHICAL ISSUES

Background

The aim of this chapter is to explore how nurses can improve their recognition of ethical issues related to their day-to-day practice and as part of the ethical reasoning process. This involves the mental health nurse becoming more ethically sensitive while at the same effectively managing the moral distress that can arise from being exposed to difficult situations. Mental health nursing practice can throw up situations that feel similar and yet can be quite unique in their own way. This uniqueness emanates from the interpersonal nature of mental health practice, meaning that the nurse has to be sensitive to common ethical issues such as consent, and at the same time unique ethical elements that are values-related (Smith 2012b; Bloch and Green 2006; Roberts 2004). On this basis this chapter will present an extended scenario that a mental health nurse could well encounter in their practice. This scenario will also be explored throughout the rest of the book as part of the ethical reasoning process.

> Michael is 35 years old and has recently split from his long-term partner. He has just moved back to his parents' home. He has a history of depressive episodes, which have been managed successfully with antidepressant medication. Michael has been offered talking therapies; however, he tried one session and did not go back as he did not really like talking about his feelings. This was the same picture when he agreed to go with his partner to relationship counselling – he again lasted only one session. Michael describes himself as a worrier; when asked about these worries he just says 'I worry about everything'.

A month ago Michael was interviewed by the police about constantly sending text messages to his ex-partner demanding to know if she is seeing someone else. The messages are not offensive, just repetitively asking the same question, around 100 times, day and night. His ex-partner does not want to get Michael into trouble she just wants the messages to stop; she has now changed her mobile number. A couple of weeks ago Michael was persuaded by his parents to go to hospital as he had admitted to them that while they were away at the weekend he had taken a large number of tablets with the intention of killing himself. On assessment by mental health crisis services Michael mentioned that he was worried about being seen by the police and he was having ruminating thoughts about being a bad person, he was not sleeping very well and he could not face eating food. He felt worthless, and he just wanted to die and end his suffering by any means. He felt conflicted by these thoughts and feelings as he knew his death would upset his parents, leaving him with a sense that he must get help. Michael could not give any guarantees that he would not try and kill himself again.

Subsequently Michael was admitted informally to an acute in-patient mental health ward, within 6 hours of arriving on the ward, Michael spoke to the nurse in charge and stated that he wanted to go home, his reasons were that the ward was too noisy and it was making him feel worse. After the nurse and the doctor assessed Michael he was put on a section of the Mental Health Act, at this juncture he became angry, shouting you ask me to be honest and then you treat me like a criminal. He then started to throw objects around and beating his fists against the wall, as staff tried to de-escalate the situation Michael ignored them and started to try and break the window by using a chair. He became frustrated that the window would not break so he threw the chair at a member of staff who sustained a head injury. On realising what he had done Michael stopped what he was doing sat down on the floor and started to cry, saying 'I am so sorry, I just wanted to go home to die.'

Structured reflection

When thinking about the scenario or any practice situation it is useful as a way of capturing initial impressions to consider the following (Shaffer and Zikmund-Fisher 2013):

- What overall message is contained within the story?
- Does the story prompt you to change your practice?
- What does the story say about how the service user was treated?
- Do you feel connected to the story, how does it make you feel?
- Is the overall tone of the story positive or negative?
- What factors could be changed to make the story feel more positive?

When re-reading the scenario I felt a sense of sadness and frustration, it felt as if Michael was trapped in a situation and I wanted to help, I wanted to talk with Michael and try and improve his situation. Let us move beyond initial impressions to consider how these thoughts and feelings can be structured in a way that learning takes place. This process is called reflection which has the following common features (Smith 2014, pp.85):

- Identify and describe the experience.
- Examine the experience in depth, tease out the key issues.
- Process the issues: how do the issues relate to practice and what have I learnt?
- In the light of examining this experience, what actions do I need to take, how can I improve my practice?

Professionally there is the expectation that the nurses regularly engage in reflection and this will be structured through the NMC's code of conduct: 'The Code will be central in the revalidation process as a focus for professional reflection. This will give the Code significance in your professional life, and raise its status and importance for employers' (NMC 2015a: 3).

There is the added expectation that reflecting on practice will enable the nurse to improve their practice and improve the quality of the care they deliver (NMC 2015a; Smith 2014). Being reflective in a way that leads to learning requires a level of criticality (Smith 2014). This can be undertaken through asking a series of questions such as the ones that follow (Crowe and O'Malley 2006):

- Why is the issue problematic?
- Why has it occurred?
- What is it impact?
- Are there alternative ways of managing the issue?
- Is there evidence available which helps?

Reflection can be post-experience, reflection on action, and it can also happen during the experience, reflection in action, as seen with expert practitioners (Smith 2014). Learning to reflect in a structured way takes time and especially where it needs to be fluid and skilled rather than being rigid like following a set formula (ibid.).

The more refined and embedded the reflective process becomes the more likely the nurse will become an expert practitioner who is skilled in reflecting in action (ibid.; Benner 1982). The scenario highlights a number of common ethical issues that mental health nurses typically encounter in their day-to-day practice; one issue I want to tease out as a reflective commentary and examine in more depth is the issue of autonomy (Roberts 2004).

Michael wants to leave the ward and prior to arriving on the ward he was openly expressing the intention that he wanted to kill himself. The nurse could have said fine you can discharge yourself, or could they? Michael has a mental health condition and has been admitted to a mental health facility for treatment, this means that the nurse as the treater has a duty of care, so what is their duty towards Michael? They need to keep him safe and provide the best treatment available, they also have to recognise that Michael may well be so disabled by his condition that he does not know what is in his best interests (NMC 2015a). To keep Michael on the ward would increase the chances of preventing harm and it would also increase the chances of treating the underlying mental disorder and therefore potentially reducing the risk of harm, an act that would do good (Roberts 2004; Beauchamp and Childress 2009; NMC 2015a).

Keeping Michael on the ward is coercive, however it is ethically justifiable not just because it is state sanctioned (duty of care) it also leads to doing good (Ripstein 2004; O'Brien and Golding 2003; NMC 2015a). This does not mean that the use of coercive measures on a routine basis are always ethically justifiable, if Michael was not a risk and he had no history or intention of harming himself, then on those grounds he should be allowed to discharge himself (O'Brien and Golding 2003). This means that each situation has to be considered individually and on its ethical merits (NMC 2015a). Using coercion even in the case of Michael being diagnosed with a mental illness, intending to commit suicide, not acting autonomously, and where the mental health nurse is professionally obligated to intervene can also be seen as being paternalistic (Beauchamp and Childress 2009). Note Michael's comment about being treated like a criminal. Paternalism is having the authority to restrict freedoms, similar to sanctioned coercion (ibid.). Within mental health nursing practice this is soft paternalism:

> In soft paternalism, an agent intervenes in the life of another person on grounds of beneficence or nonmaleficence with the goal of preventing sub-stantially nonvoluntary conduct. Substantially nonvoluntary actions include cases such as poor informed consent or refusal, severe depression that precludes rational deliberation and addiction that prevents free choice and action.
>
> *(Beauchamp and Childress 2009: 209–210)*

Whereas hard paternalism 'by contrast, involves interventions intended to prevent or mitigate harm to or to benefit a person, despite the fact that the person's risky choices and actions are informed, voluntary, and autonomous' (ibid.).

Irrespective of the difference in the definitions Michael feels angry, he is being stopped from doing want he wants irrelevant of how irrational his thinking is at that moment in time. Michael is unable to govern his actions to a point where he is putting himself and others at risk and on this basis the nurse has to govern and control Michael in a way that is proportional to the harm it is preventing (Roberts 2004; Liégeois and Eneman 2008). Interestingly someone was harmed by Michael's actions, should the nurse have acted sooner? This is something we will explore further in the next section.

Clinical supervision

The Care Quality Commission (CQC) describes three types of supervision and their corresponding features within health and social care settings:

1 Managerial supervision is delivered by a staff member's manager it focuses on:
   - Reviewing performance
   - Setting priorities that are in line with the service need
   - Identifying continuing development needs
2 Clinical supervision provides time for a member of staff to:
   - Reflect on and review their practice
   - Discuss individual cases
   - Change their practice
   - Identify continuing development needs
3 Professional supervision is like clinical supervision, however the supervisor is from the same profession:
   - Reflect on and review their practice in line with professional standards
   - Discuss individual cases in line with professional standards
   - Identify continuing development needs in line with professional standards

(Care Quality Commission 2013: 3–4)

Mental health nurses will receive managerial supervision in addition they may also access clinical supervision which will and should have the features of professional supervision, the difference being that they may not also be supervised by a nurse. The NMC (2006) recognises the importance of clinical supervision in terms of providing a protected space where the nurse can reflect on their practice, improve the quality of their practice and identify their continuing professional development needs (ibid.). This practice should be framed by the NMC's standards for professional conduct and continuing professional development (ibid.). The NMC does not state which model of clinical supervision a nurse should follow instead they suggest this practice should be framed by the following set of principles:

- Clinical supervision supports practice, enabling registrants to maintain and improve standards of care.
- Clinical supervision is a practice-focused professional relationship, involving a practitioner reflecting on practice guided by a skilled supervisor.
- Registrants and managers should develop the process of clinical supervision according to local circumstances. Ground rules should be agreed so that the supervisor and the registrant approach clinical supervision openly, confidently and are aware of what is involved.

- Every registrant should have access to clinical supervision and each supervisor should supervise a realistic number of practitioners.
- Preparation for supervisors should be flexible and sensitive to local circumstances. The principles and relevance of clinical supervision should be included in pre-registration and post-registration education programmes
- Evaluation of clinical supervision is needed to assess how it influences care and practice standards. Evaluation systems should be determined locally.

(NMC 2006: 1–2)

Clinical supervision can be delivered as individual supervision or through group supervision, the challenge for the nurse who is accessing either group or individual supervision is to make sure it meets their professional needs (Smith 2014; NMC 2006). Engaging in clinical supervision provides structured time in which the nurse can critically reflect on their practice with the long-term benefits (Care Quality Commission 2013) of:

- improving the standard of care they delivered;
- assisting them to develop effective ways of managing the emotional dimension of practice;
- improving job satisfaction and staff retention;
- improving how risks are managed;
- promoting good practice; and
- systematically identifying continuing development needs.

To be effective clinical supervision needs to be structured, it also needs to have a formal contract (Freshwater 2011). This contract which is agreed between the supervisor and the subordinate will set the ground rules which include agreeing on the number of sessions, the responsibilities of both parties, how records are kept and stored, the model used, and how confidentiality is manged (ibid.). The structure of the sessions will be shaped by the reflective model the supervisor and subordinate agree to use, however most models will following a common process, identifying the issues to be addressed, critically examining these issues in depth, setting agreed actions to be addressed, and evaluating these actions (ibid.). This process can be fluid depending on what the issue is, the subordinate may find that an issue is discussed many times and that just because it goes through a structured process it does not mean it is resolved there and then especially when dealing with the emotional context of practice (ibid.; Gardner 2014). Most times, and certainly within mental health nursing practice, ethical issues will reside within that emotional psychosocial realm, as very rarely will the mental health nurse be dealing with the bioethics issues of abortion, euthanasia to name a few (Gardner 2014; Holt and Convey 2012). Mental health nurses will deal with issues that are more pervasive and, values-based, and ethically conflicting (Holt and Convey 2012). This conflict can be external; it can also be internalised leading to ethical distress (ibid.).

As a reflective commentary let us explore 'should the nurse have acted sooner'. When talking to her colleagues, the nurse in charge of the situation was reassured that she did everything that she could, in other words she did the right thing, however she does not feel she did the right thing (ibid.). This feeling was based on the outcome that her colleague was injured, the nurse wonders whether she could have prevented this happening. She felt by giving Michael as much time, using restraint as a last option, that she was setting up the conditions to de-escalate the situation and yet at the point Michael picked up the chair she realised she was no longer in control of the situation (Smith 2014). The nurse decided to take this issue to her next clinical supervision session (Holt and Convey 2012). During the session the nurse explored this issue and started to recognise that she had conflicting duties, her duty to Michael and her duty to her colleagues. By giving Michael as much time as possible the nurse felt she had discharged her duty to Michael and yet Michael was distressed by his actions, so she was not entirely sure. The member of staff who was injured spoke to the nurse after the incident did not blame her, 'it's part of the job', she felt this should not be the case. Considering other options the nurse recognised that if the team had tried to restrain Michael before he picked up the chair this would have been wrong, as it was not proportionate and if they had tried to restrain Michael when he had the chair in hand more people could have been injured. During this reflective process the nurse started to feel less distressed (Edwards *et al.* 2006; Begat *et al.* 2005; de Veer *et al.* 2013).

Working with the service user narrative

Using clinical supervision to engage a critical dialogue can help to effectively manage a mental health nurse's emotional and ethical distress that arises from their practice, however it is important to recognise that the service user is missing from this process (Gardner 2014). Even though Michael was not restrained, however there was a restrictive element present during the incident the National Institute for Clinical Excellence (NICE) suggests:

> After using a restrictive intervention, and when the risks of harm have been contained, conduct an immediate post-incident debrief, including a nurse and a doctor, to identify and address physical harm to service users or staff, ongoing risks and the emotional impact on service users and staff, including witnesses.
>
> *(NICE 2015: 37)*

During this process Michael should have the opportunity to discuss the incident in a supportive way, an advocate should be present, and Michael should also be given the opportunity to write about his thoughts and feelings (ibid.). In addition there should be a more formal de-briefing which should:

- Be undertaken no later than 72 hours after the incident.
- Be undertaken by a team of trained investigators from outside the ward.
- Use information recorded in the immediate debrief, the service user's notes relating to the incident, and the interviews with the staff, Michael, and witnesses.
- Evaluate the physical and emotional impact of the incident on all parties who were involved.
- Consider if things could have been done differently and/or less restrictive.
- Determine if there are barriers which make it difficult to avoid the same course of action happening in the future.
- Recommend changes where appropriate.
- Provide a formal report of the team's findings to the ward (ibid.).

This process involves on-going dialogue with Michael where Michael is listened to, this dialogue needs to be located within the therapeutic relationship, and it also needs to drive the process of planning and delivering care (Chambers *et al.* 2014). Even though the staff team have been through a difficult situation with Michael they still need to have a positive attitude; 'Building and establishing effective and trusting relationships with service users promotes and supports recovery and enables involvement and control over their 'conditions', treatment and care' (ibid.: 6).

The therapeutic relationship is so important especially as this relationship is the medium for treatment as well as in most cases the main treatment (Radden 2002; Smith 2014). The nurse knows that all parties involved in the incident are distressed by what has happened; as the nurse has a duty of care to Michael she then has to facilitate a way forward that helps Michael resolve this distress in a way that ultimately helps him to recover (Chambers *et al.* 2014).

The de-briefing process provides a framework in which to structure what at times can be a difficult conversation for all parties, however by focusing on the need to learn this conversation should be positive and solution focused (NICE 2015). Being positive and ultimately recovery-focused should be part and parcel of the therapeutic relationship as should being open, honest and also person-centred (Smith 2014). By taking this approach a therapeutic alliance is created which is a true partnership and gives the latitude to fully explore ethical issues that are specific to mental health nursing practice such as the use of coercion (Perraud *et al.* 2006; Wilkin 2006; Roberts 2004). Returning to Michael, let us consider how this relationship works in practice.

After the incident Michael's primary nurse Michelle recognises that there is a need to start building a therapeutic relationship with Michael and his family. Michael was only on the ward for a short period of time before the incident, so he had not had the opportunity to really connect with any of the staff on the ward. To start building this relationship Michelle was empathetic, actively listening to Michael's experiences, being person-centred by accepting the person, and showing care and compassion at what is a difficult time for Michael (Smith 2014). At the same time as managing the emotional dimension of the therapeutic relationship Michelle was reasoning through the next steps and developing a plan of care that would be evidenced-based. At the moment Michelle was reasoning that as a priority Michael needed to be kept safe; some measures would be short-term while Michelle worked with Michael to develop more healthy and sustainable ways of coping (Chambers *et al.* 2014). During this process Michelle would have to potentially make difficult emotional decisions which will have an ethical component such as balancing the need to respect Michael's autonomy against the need to keep Michael safe which may mean that Michael's freedoms are temporally restricted (Roberts 2004; Bloch and Green 2006). As Michael recovers the expectation is that he will self-manage his risk by developing healthy ways of coping with his mental distress such as being mindful when he has ruminating thoughts (Smith 2014). Dealing with ethical conflict Michelle knows she has to be emotionally responsive to how Michael and his family feel about any proposed course of action while recognising Michael's current vulnerability; Michael due to his mental distress may find it difficult to make a reasoned decision (Roberts 2004).

To be emotionally responsive Michelle has to be empathetic and self-aware. Sometimes this does not happen as mental health nurses do not always pay full attention to the service user's point of view (Smith 2012a). Michael mentioned during the incident that he felt he was being treated like a criminal; this is a powerful statement which contains a potent emotional message (Martinez 2009). It would be easy for Michelle to reconstruct this as Michael not understanding what is going on and once he is well he will understand that everything was done in his best interests (Merleau–Ponty 1945/1962; Bracken and Thomas 2005; Berlin 1998/2000). If this happens this would be a missed opportunity to help Michael and Michele to make sense of their shared experiences:

> Relationships are co-constructed, and the experience of the service user depends on what happens between him or her and the professional. The mutual validation and consciousness of sharing the same mental landscape may reaffirm experience of belonging with others in society…
>
> *(Ådnøy Eriksen 2014: 111)*

To maximise this opportunity Michelle has to facilitate Michael to talk about his experiences in a way that is non-directive and does not reinterpret Michael's experiences (ibid.).

A two-way dialogue

To be sensitive to Michael's story Michelle has to possess certain character traits, as a nurse these would include being (NMC 2015a):

- kind;
- respectful;
- compassionate;
- polite;
- supportive;
- honest;
- reflective; and
- competent.

Within mental health nursing practice these traits have to be fully utilised throughout the therapeutic relationship; 'To be effective, such relationships need to be therapeutic in nature, encompassing an emotional human interaction' (McAndrew *et al.* 2014: 213).

To build an effective therapeutic relationship the nurse has to engender trust, this can be a challenge due to the controlling nature of mental health nursing practice. Dinç and Gastermans (2013) identified trust within a generic nursing context as something that is highly valued by service users. To engender trust the nurse has to be a competent practitioner, they have to be available and accessible, they have to be informative, and have a good attitude and manner (ibid.). It is important to note that trust within the therapeutic relationship:

- is a dynamic and on-going process;
- evolves with the relationship;
- is person-centred; and
- can be easily broken (ibid.).

Depersonalising the service user can lead to trust being broken, which includes not viewing the service user as a person first (ibid.). In addition, mental health service users 'considered values and attitudes to be more important than technical skills' (McAndrew *et al.* 2014: 215).

The challenge for Michelle is that the vehicle for conveying the right values and attitudes is through listening and talking, activities that are not always prioritised on acute mental health wards (ibid.). This means that Michelle has to make an effort to spend time with Michael; this is not about spending lots of time with Michael it is about spending quality time with Michael (ibid.). Michael telling his story can be a healing process, however; 'The narration of personal stories will only occur if a service user is given time, safe space, and encouragement to tell' (ibid.: 214).

During this time of facilitating Michael to tell his story there is a duty of care to manage risk. Michael telling his story will have an emotional depth one that he has difficulty in coping healthily with; this may mean that the risk of Michael harming himself increases. Preventing harm is crucial and part of Michelle's role, at this juncture coercive strategies may have to be used (Beauchamp and Childress 2009; O'Brien and Golding 2003). Of course Michelle should always follow the least coercive approach where using a coercive strategy. O'Brien and Golding (ibid.) highlight it is better if 'harm caused by coercion is much less than the harm caused by the action they would have chosen if left uncoerced' (ibid.: 172). On this basis Michelle has to make a judgement that is being coercive right for Michael at that moment in time. The implication of this is that Michelle has to be sensitive to the individual nature of a situation to ensure that the coercion will benefit Michael.

Mental health nurses generally have to be sensitive to the individual context of care by being able to quickly respond and in the right way. It would be easy to say responding in the right way is just about logic and evidence-base but as 'caring' professionals nurses also have to respond at an emotional level, which means that nurses have to be emotionally sensitive (Smith 2012a). The main way that nurses can be seen to be emotionally sensitive as a good thing is through the use of character traits and through knowing the service user they are working with (Armstrong 2006; Roberts 2004). Being sensitive at an emotional level is not just about character traits it also about making the right decision at the right time (Radden 2002). Michelle should treat Michael with respect and in the process focus on building a sustainable therapeutic relationship that will also preserve Michael's ethical dignity (Bloch and Green 2006). Knowing Michael will help Michelle when working in the complex nature of mental health nursing practice to be morally sensitive and morally responsive, it will also help Michelle to utilise the right character traits at the right time (Bloch and Green 2006).How do you know whether a mental nurse has the right character traits? Let us return to the scenario:

> Being empathetic is a key factor in working effectively with Michael, a view that is endorsed by a community of practice, and on this basis the mental health nurse would need to cultivate empathetic character traits (Radden and Sadler 2008; McAndrew *et al.* 2014). Michelle as the treater in the therapeutic relationship should adopt and develop certain character traits or virtues, but these character traits do not sit in isolation as the mental health nursing community of practice clearly identifies what character traits a mental health nurse should adopt to be an effective treater (Roberts 2004; NMC 2015a). Empathy is a key trait, one that will help Michelle to engender trust and establish a two-way dialogue where Michael's story becomes part of his journey towards recovery (Bracken and Thomas 2005). Michelle works with Michael's story by not taking a segmented approach and listens to the whole of the story as if afresh (Smith 2012a; Bracken and Thomas 2005). This gives Michelle the opportunity to explore multiple meanings within the story,

such as what does 'being locked up like a criminal' feel like from Michael's perspective (Bracken and Thomas 2005). By Michael re-telling his story and working with different elements of the story this can in itself be a medium for healing (ibid.).

Key learning points

1 To recognise ethical issues the mental health nurse has to be ethically sensitive. They also have to be aware of any moral distress in the most difficult situations.

2 When considering a practice situation, a useful way of capturing initial impressions is to consider the overall message of the situation. Are there things the nurse can learn? Is there an emotional dimension to the situation? If so, what is it? How does the situation link to the notion of recovery?

3 Building on initial impressions the nurse can then move onto the reflective process, identify and describe the experience, examine the experience in depth, process the issues, and consider how practice can be improved.

4 Professionally there is the expectation that the nurses regularly engage in reflection and this will be structured through the NMC's (2015a) code of conduct.

5 The Care Quality Commission (2013) describes three types of supervision: managerial supervision, clinical supervision, professional supervision.

6 Mental health nurses will be managerially supervised, they may also in addition access clinical supervision which will and should have the features of professional supervision, the difference being that they may not also be supervised by a nurse. Clinical supervision provides a protected space where the nurse can reflect on their practice, improve the quality of their practice and identify their continuing professional development needs. This practice should be framed by the NMC's standards for professional conduct and continuing professional development (NMC 2015b).

7 Using clinical supervision to engage in a critical dialogue can help to effectively manage a mental health nurse's emotional and ethical distress that arises from their practice. However it is important to recognise that the service user is missing from this process. During this process the service user should have the opportunity to discuss the incident in a supportive way, an advocate should be present, and the service user should also be given the opportunity to write about their thoughts and feelings.

8 The formal de-briefing process provides a framework in which to structure what at times can be a difficult conversation for all parties, however by focusing on the need to learn this conversation should be positive and solution focused.

9 To be sensitive to the service user's story the nurse has to possess certain character traits; within mental health nursing practice these traits have to be fully utilised within the therapeutic relationship.

10 To build an effective therapeutic relationship the nurse has to engender trust which can be a challenge due to the controlling nature of mental health nursing practice. Trust is highly valued by service users. To engender trust the nurse has to be a competent practitioner, they have to be available and accessible, they have to be informative, and a have good attitude and manner.

5
GATHERING FACTS AND VALUES

Background

This chapter will explore how mental health nurses gather facts and values, and how this information can be used as part of the ethical reasoning process. A key part of gathering this information is the assessment process. However, this information can create ethical conflict, so we will also explore how this conflict can be managed through a good process, something we explored briefly in Chapter 3. Collecting information or evidence has in recent years been heavily influenced by the drive towards clinical effectiveness (Newell and Gournay 2009). This drive within mental health nursing can be traced back to the advent of evidenced-based medicine within psychiatry. Gournay in 1995 was articulating the view that mental health nursing practice should only be based on theories that are testable and have reliability (Gournay 1995). By taking this view Gournay was trying to move mental health nursing away from using nursing models and towards using evidence derived ideally from randomised control trials. Gournay (ibid.) gave an example of how this would work in practice, and has subsequently written a number of papers and resources articulating what evidence-based mental health nursing should look like (Newell and Gournay 2009). Interestingly this approach only indicates the types of evidence the nurse should use, it does not provide examples of how this approach works in unstructured and unplanned situations and where scientific evidence is not available (ibid.).

Fundamentally Gournay (1995) was dismissing the value of all other knowledge that is not evidence-based knowledge or scientific knowledge. This view is based on the notion that only logical and objective approaches can help mental health nurses make sense of their practice (Franks 2004). Franks provides a challenge to this view on the premise that scientific evidence cannot provide the only truth or viewpoint (ibid.). Returning to Michael and Michelle, introduced in Chapter 4, a good example of different viewpoints is the way risk is quantified. To collect clinical risk information about Michael and his circumstances Michelle will use a risk assessment tool which has been designed specifically to collect quantifiable information with the intention of assisting in the prediction and subsequent management of clinical risk (Smith 2014; Rylance and Simpson 2012). One of the limitations with this empiric approach is that a score could not have predicted the way Michael reacted when he felt frustrated. In addition, when Michelle tries to capture the outcome of this situation, can a score really suffice? Was Michael violent or was it an accident? This sort of uncertainty is why assessing clinical risk requires more information than a score; it also requires a narrative (Smith 2012a; Rylance and Simpson 2012).

Similar to the move towards evidence-based practice there has been a move to ensure ethical reasoning rules are also objective (McCarthy 2003). This has been influenced by the ethical approach called principlism that has dominated bioethics especially within the medical field for a number of years, we will explore this approach in more depth within the Chapter 6 (ibid.). The perceived attractiveness of principlism is that it is seen as less difficult to use than other moral theories and therefore more useful as an ethical reasoning framework, it also has a clinical emphasis (Callahan 2003; Smith Iltis 2000). Principlism can be seen as a straightforward way of making ethical clinical decisions even in complex situations (Callahan 2003). According to Edwards (2009) the key advantages of using principlism within the field of nursing is that principlism is easily applied to the vast majority of ethical problems faced by nurses. However, according to McCarthy (2006), one of the key problems with principlism is that as a generic framework it does not acknowledge the unique issues and practices that can arise. One such issue in mental health nursing practice is the issue of coercion and the power that the mental health nurse can hold over a service user (Roberts 2004). The rest of this chapter will explore how mental health nurses can collect information that is inclusive and reason in a way that is also inclusive.

The assessment process

Gathering information through assessment is an important part of mental health nursing practice, it is an activity that is never-ending as mental health nurses constantly collect service user information (Coombs *et al.* 2011). Mental health nurses will collect a wide range of information throughout a service user's care journey, other professionals, the service user, and carers will also collect and add their information to the information the mental nurse has collected (Smith 2014). The information the nurse collects should be comprehensive, giving the nurse a full picture of the service user and how they are functioning, and it will include information on their; physical health, psychological and social functioning, and their spiritual needs (ibid.).

Once collected assessment information will be used as part of the care planning and care delivery process:

It assists the mental health nurse and service user in partnership to identify what the issues are and what needs to be addressed. The next step is to consider as a partnership is what we are trying to achieve, what changes would we like to take place and by when. After this step the partnership would consider what interventions would be the most useful, also at this stage the relevant clinical guidelines would need to be taken into consideration. Finally did we achieve our goals, if not why not, is there another approach we could consider?

(Smith 2014: 25)

The assessment process to be effective has to be collaborative; it also has to be underpinned by the appropriate use of both verbal and non-verbal communication skills (Knott 2012; Smith 2014). This process also has to be goal-focused, what information do you need to collect and why? Curran and Rogers (2004: 9) suggest that to be comprehensive the assessment process needs to focus on collecting the following information:

- detailed information about the presenting problem;
- a clear description about the service user's mental distress;
- risk factors and protective factors;
- social and occupational function;
- support networks; and
- carer's perspective.

To collect this information the mental health nurse will use a variety of methods which will include; asking questions, recording what they observe, and rating behaviours and symptoms (Smith 2014). Asking questions will lead to the rating of behaviours and symptoms and during this process the nurse will observe the service user's behaviour (Curran and Rogers 2004). The challenge is to ask the right questions! Curran and Rogers suggest the mental health nurse starts with open questions which will give broad information, they then move onto more leading or probing questions as they focus on specific areas, and then will use closed questions to give more detail within those specific areas (ibid.). This process can be shaped by the use of assessment tools where a nurse may start with a tool that looks at the general functioning of the service user and finishes with the use of a tool that focuses on a specific issue such as hearing voices (Smith 2014). For example when Michael was admitted to the ward a general assessment would have been completed before admission; this information would have been built on during the admission process by both the psychiatrist and the admitting mental health nurse. In addition specific questions would have been asked about risk and about his symptoms, this process is usually framed by a number of assessment tools.

Mental health nurses will investigate a number of areas during the assessment process; this will include identifying the problem with a focus on helping the service user to find solutions to the problem (Coombs *et al.* 2011). This approach fits in with the care planning process; however finding solutions that are sustainable is dependent on the nurse building an effective therapeutic relationship (Smith 2014). Relationship building will start during the assessment phase where a rapport is established and a plan of care is agreed (Coombs *et al.* 2011). One key area that the mental health nurse will focus on is the assessment of risk (Coombs *et al.* 2013). Clinical risk for mental health nurses is about the need to predict whether a client may harm themselves and/or others (Smith 2014). Information related to risk is collected and made sense of in different ways as nurses will use different forms of knowledge (see Chapter 2). Based on the seminal work of Carper (1978) ways of knowing about a service user's risk is discovered in the following ways:

1 Empiric knowing – risk is understood through the use of validated risk assessment tools which categorise risk.
2 Aesthetic knowing – risk is understood through the service user's unique story, their narrative.
3 Personal knowing – risk is understood through the therapeutic relationship where the mental health nurse knows the service user through being self-aware and being empathetic.
4 Ethical knowing – risk is understood through the mental health nurse being sensitive to that service user's values and constantly balancing the service user's values against the nurse's professional duties.

Assessing risk is the first stage in managing risk, this is not a segmented process rather it is a dynamic process of continually assessing and managing risk within the multi-disciplinary team which fits in with the best practice of structured risk assessment where all forms of knowing are actively used (Rylance and Simpson 2012; Carper 1978). The types of risk information the mental health nurse will routinely collect include (Rylance and Simpson 2012):

• historical – family, mental health, social, employment, medical and risk;
• mental state and drug screening;
• staff observations and self-reported information;
• risk triggers;
• cooperation with treatment;
• symptoms; and
• protective factors.

Mental health nursing is heavily influenced by evidence-based practice so there is the tendency to focus on this type of evidence rather than take a more rounded approach (Morgan *et al.* 2016; Barker 2001). To ensure that the values element is not missing during the assessment process which includes assessing risk, the process has to be person-centred, it has to takes all perspectives into account, and it should also consider the strengths of the service user (Morgan *et al.* 2016; Coombs *et al.* 2013; Wand 2011). At this point we return to Michael.

Michelle realised that the risk assessment process did not fully explain that Michael can become angry and impulsive when frustrated. Michelle was also interested in why this did not happen all the time. Michelle decided to explore with Michael such issues and what prevents Michael acting in this way, how he controls his behaviour, and what triggers this behaviour.

Values to facts

The facts or values debate came to prominence in the 1960s led by the work of Thomas Szasz who focused on the objectivity of mental illness;

> Mental illness, of course, is not literally a 'thing' – or physical object – and hence it can 'exist' only in the same sort of way in which other theoretical concepts exist. Yet, familiar theories are in the habit of posing, sooner or later... as 'objective truths' (or 'facts').
>
> *(Szasz 1960: 113)*

Szasz went on to talk about the myth of mental illness, not everyone will agree with his viewpoint, however as Kendall articulates:

> although his core arguments have not, broadly speaking, been accepted, he has made many psychiatrists, social scientists, and jurists think about issues they might not otherwise have considered and key assumptions they might never have questioned.
>
> *(Kendell 2004: 46)*

Questioning key assumptions about the nature of mental illness has led to the position that facts and values cannot always be easily separated and what appears to be a fact may indeed be a value (Fulford 2004). For example a mental health nurse may read a service user's psychiatric assessment which indicates that the service user has a mental illness, say depression, this may appear to be a fact because it has gone through a scientific process, or is it a value that looks like a fact? The use of diagnostic criteria has changed over time, some would say evolved. Diagnosis or applying a diagnostic label some might say is more robust, however this process of applying a label is still dependent on the judgement of the observer (ibid.).

Fulford *et al.* make the following point:

> The traditional medical model, then, rests on the idea that, however crucial values may be in other areas of health care, diagnosis is a 'purely' scientific exercise. In psychiatry this amounts to the claim that psychopathology

(symptoms) and the classification (of disorders), on which the process of diagnosis depends, must all be value free.

(Fulford et al. *2006: 565)*

The attraction to understanding a service user's experience of mental distress as a 'purely scientific exercise' or evidence-based approach using criteria and tools is that it appears to all intents and purposes values free (ibid.). The use of scientific terminology in Michael's case, depression, infers there something happening to Michael that can be objectively interpreted by an adequately trained other person and both parties would agree that Michael has a mental illness called depression (Bracken and Thomas 2005; Feely *et al.* 2007). The use of an agreed classification framework should make this process robust, however depression cannot be seen under a microscope like a disease process, it is seen through being self-reported, observed and then an interpretative judgement is made, therefore it cannot escape being contextualised by values (Boorse 1975; Fulford *et al.* 2006). Michael defines himself as a worrier – a value judgement. Once he has entered services, being a worrier has now become 'Michael has depression', which feels like a fact.

For worrying to become a diagnosis of depression, at least two of the three core symptoms are present every day for two weeks:

* low mood;
* loss of interest; and
* low energy (Smith 2014).

Associated symptoms include:

* disturbed sleep;
* poor concentration;
* low self-confidence;
* poor appetite;
* suicidal thoughts or acts;
* agitation;
* slowing of movements; and
* guilt.

To establish Michael has depression, the psychiatrist along with other members of the multi-disciplinary team will interpret Michael's story and reported behaviours and then they will compare it to the classification criteria for depression (Fulford *et al.* 2006). This in itself creates a circular process where Michael's story and behaviours lead to a diagnosis of depression. These behaviours are then seen as symptoms of depression, having symptoms of depression then means that Michael has depression. Pathologising Michael's behaviour and story then leads to how Michael's behaviours are managed; his symptoms of depression. Michael has tried to kill himself, he has a diagnosis of depression; this will be seen as a symptom of his condition (Redfield Jamison 2000). Again, the circular argument comes into play if Michael had successfully killed himself without being diagnosed with depression it would be highly likely on reviewing his case history that it would be inferred that he had undiagnosed depression (ibid.). The implication being that if you treat depression you will reduce the symptoms of depression including the risk of suicide (Antai-Otong 2003).

Having this label of depression, which is a value turned into a fact through an agreed criteria, can create an added layer of values. Chur-Hansen *et al.* (2005) provide a good example of this in action, making the point that mental health nurses are optimistic about the prognosis of someone who has been diagnosed with depression. However this optimism is dependent on the a number of factors being present:

- The service user engages in treatment and this treatment is provided in the early stages of the condition.
- The service user has supportive social circumstances.
- The service user was functioning at a good level before they became 'ill'.
- The service user did have a history of drug use, post-traumatic stress disorder, bipolar illness, childhood sexual abuse, unresolved grief, or difficult childhood, suicidality.

Ethical conflict

This need to turn values into facts can create conflict especially if we look at the area of evidence-based practice (Wand 2011). This approach generalises experience so Michael's worrying behaviour becomes depression after being processed through an internationally agreed criteria (ibid.). This means that Michael's depression will have common features with other people's experience of depression, however how Michael makes sense of his experience of depression is unique to Michael (Barker 2001; Wand 2011). There is a need to have a shared language and using agreed terms like depression which can be useful especially for research and treatment purposes, the nurse also needs to acknowledge that using the term depression provides only one version of the 'truth' (Fulford *et al.* 2006). To understand Michael's experiences of his mental distress Michelle has to move beyond the use of a diagnostic term. Understanding or even trying to understand someone else's experience of mental distress can be a challenge, we experience our lives in a fluid way and sometimes it is difficult to find the words to explain what is happening (Varelius 2009). Returning to Michael and the scenario, let us consider some key experiences:

- Relationship ending
- History of mental distress
- Prefers medication than therapy
- Not comfortable with sharing his feelings

- Tries to talk about his feelings
- Worries a lot
- Does not always understand the impact of actions upon others
- Wants to kill himself
- Ruminating thoughts
- Will talk to his parents
- Not sleeping
- Not eating
- Does not value himself
- Does not want to upset people
- Death would end his suffering
- Dislikes noise
- Angry
- Tries not to hurt others
- Prefers being at home

This list is my interpretation of Michael's story; there may be others. The next step is to check with Michael not that the list is right but that the list has a shared sense of meaning (Fulford *et al.* 2006). Once this shared sense of meaning is established this provides the opportunity to probe further and for Michelle to explore other truths not fully uncovered by the risk assessment process:

- when Michael is frustrated he can become angry and impulsive, but not all the time;
- what triggers these behaviours; and
- what prevents this behaviour happening more often.

It is important to note that most of time Michael's coping strategies have worked until recently, his mental distress appears to be a signal that he is not coping and that this is a negative experience for Michael (Fulford *et al.* 2006). Also focusing on what works for Michael, Michelle is moving away from a one-size-fits-all approach and is considering wellbeing, what keeps Michael well and what does well look like for Michael, a more positive approach (Wand 2011; Barker 2001). This approach is pragmatic and recovery-based, it is shaped by the real world, and it reflects Michael's wants, needs, experiences and aspirations (Barker 2001).

Being pragmatic creates further challenges. Michael wants to go home, he does not like the noise on the ward, and he still wants to die. The challenge for Michelle is does she allow Michael to go home, where he wants to be, and run the risk of Michael killing himself, or keep Michael on the ward where she has more control over him, knowing that he feels more unwell on the ward and extremely frustrated (Hall 2004)? If we look at the facts (values into facts), Michael has been diagnosed with depression, he wants to kill himself, he does not want to remain on the ward and is actively trying to leave. It looks fairly straightforward, Michelle, as part of the ward team could use a section of the mental health act to detain Michael, so he is not going anywhere; and yet Michael would feel this would breach his auto-nomy: 'you are treating me like a criminal'. Michelle would argue it does not as Michael is not acting autonomously, his rational thinking is disrupted by his depression and she needs to act in his best interests which at this time is to keep him on the ward (Beauchamp and Childress 2009). Within this best interests argument is the notion that Michael is being benefited and if he was in his right mind (rational) he would understand that this indeed is the case (Berlin 1998/2000, 2000; Anderson and Lux 2005). At that moment in time Michael feels controlled, using the term criminal, giving a sense that he feels he is being unfairly treated, these are values which Michelle will need to deal with as points of ethical conflict, Michelle believes she is doing the right thing, Michael believes Michelle is doing the wrong thing.

Even though Michelle can and needs to justify her actions it does not mean that by explaining her actions to Michael it will necessarily lessen his sense of being treated wrongly (Chodoff 2009; Peele and Chodoff 2009). As mental health nursing focuses heavily on the building of therapeutic relationships which have to be emotionally responsive this means that ethical decision-making within the context of this relationship is not just about reason, emotions and values play a vital part (Roberts 2004). This means that Michaels's possible sense of injustice will need to be managed and any subsequent conflict will need to be resolved, this does not mean Michelle just persuading Michael to agree with her. The first stage is to gather values, not just facts:

> People's values differ enormously – what may be important to one individual may be of little significance to another. In order to work towards good practice in mental health care it is necessary to understand the importance of the role of values.
>
> *(Woodbridge and Fulford 2004: 7)*

This process has to be an open process, one where Michelle focuses on listening and accepting that:

- values come in many varieties;
- values vary with time and place; and
- values vary from person to person (ibid.: 14–15).

Michael may not just value rights and rules, he will value having time and space, a place not being too noisy and also a sense of freedom (ibid.).

Values-based practice

Making sense of your own values is difficult enough without trying to understand someone else's values and with an eye on agreeing a way forward (Woodbridge and Fulford 2004). When exploring values there is a tendency to disagree as values can be quite personal, in addition when dealing with a difficult situation there is the tendency to determine who is right or convince the other person that your view is right (ibid.). This is a pressure that in Michael's case Michelle will feel under as the professional code of conduct among other rules based systems recommends the right values (ibid.). In this case it is important that Michelle respects Michael's values while at the same being clear that her actions are at times determined by codified rights and wrongs (ibid.).

To help practitioners like Michelle work through these challenges, Woodbridge and Fulford in their *Whose Values?* workbook suggest the mental health practitioner follow a good process called values-based practice:

> Totalitarian regimes seek to prescribe 'right' values and to make everyone work to them. This can start out with the best of intentions. Communism started out with the intention of giving everyone freedom. But in practice, 'right' values, if imposed from above, always end up becoming hardened and distorted into ideologies. In a democracy, by contrast, the principle of respect for all voices, although vulnerable in other ways (it can be hijacked by pressure groups, for example), means that there is a constant process of balancing, in order to avoid any one interest or perspective becoming too dominant. Like a political democracy, and unlike a dictatorship, values-based practice relies on 'good process' to achieve a balance of values in health care decision making.
>
> *(Woodbridge and Fulford 2004: 17)*

This process is divided into four main areas, which are then sub-divided into a number of key points. This process is summarised below using Michael's situation as an example (ibid.: 20):

- Practice skills
    1. Awareness – carefully identifying and understanding Michael's values
    2. Reasoning – clearly explaining to Michael the decision-making process that was used and what rules influenced this process
    3. Knowledge – Discussing what was known about the situation and Michael and how this influenced the decisions that were made
    4. Communication – effectively communicating throughout the awareness, reasoning, and knowledge stages
- Models of service delivery
    5. User-centred – Michael's values are the first source of information to be explored
    6. Multi-disciplinary – any outcome needs to be a balanced against all parties' perspectives
- VBP and EBP
    7. The 'two-feet' principle" – Michelle will need to recognise the decision-making process must be based on facts and values working together

8   The 'squeaky wheel' principle: Michelle will tend to recognise Michaels values when there is conflict

9   Science and values – Michelle will need to be aware that the use of scientific knowledge will potentially create a whole new set of values

- Partnership

10   Partnership – in values-based practice Michelle and Michael will need to strive towards making decisions in partnership

The strength of using a values-based approach is that it assists the nurse to manage ethical conflict in way that is collaborative and recovery-focused (Smith 2014). Values-based practice is not anti-rules or anti-science it recognises that rules and science have an important part to play in mental health nursing practice, however rules and science are not values-free and therefore values need also to be addressed (Woodbridge and Fulford 2004). If values are ignored this can create a lack of trust within the therapeutic relationship; 'VBP seeks to rebuild trust through shared decision making in which evidence and values, science and individual human needs, are equal partners' (ibid.: 32).

Values-based practice will afford Michelle the opportunity to not only reflect and explore her values but also to consider Michael's viewpoint. What does it feel like to be frustrated and have your freedoms taken away. Michelle's viewpoint may well be that protecting Michael is a good thing to do, using the practice skills highlighted in this approach Michelle can start to consider, irrelevant of how right Michelle is, Michael's viewpoint (Smith 2012b; Fulford 2009). This process does offer an added dimension to an ethical reasoning approach as values are not always considered, rather there is overwhelming focus on the facts (Fulford 2009).

In Chapter 3 there is an overview of the ethical reasoning approach used in this book and an example how the values-based approach fits within this model. Let us consider this in more detail in relation to the scenario.

Michelle has identified the main ethical issue through listening to Michael's story. There is ethical conflict due to Michelle's duty of care, keeping Michael safe, and Michael's sense of autonomy, wanting to feel he is in control and his freedom of movement is not restricted. Michelle feels that she acted in the right manner, the rules indicate that she has a duty of care and based on the facts keeping Michael on the ward is the best course of action. When reviewing the care of Michael in the ward's weekly multi-disciplinary meeting, other members of the team confirm that they believed it was the right decision. Michael is still angry about the decision and feels he has been treated unfairly. On this basis Michelle decides to meet with Michael to resolve this issue using a values-based approach, specifically the practice skills element. During this meeting Michelle considers Michael's perspective and agrees that the ward need to address his lack of freedom while at the same time keeping Michael safe. Michelle explains to Michael the influence that the law and the code of conduct have upon the decision that was made; however, Michelle accepts that there is a duty to help Michael resolve his frustrations over the incident. Michael accepts that to the 'system' it is the right decision, and yet it felt wrong. He then wanted to know how Michelle was going to help him. They both agreed a plan of action based on giving Michael more time and space as he works towards managing his risk.

Key learning points

1 Gathering both facts and values is an important part of the ethical reasoning process. This information is gathered through the ongoing assessment process; however, this information can create ethical conflict.

2 Collecting information or evidence through the assessment process has in recent years been heavily influenced by the drive towards clinical effectiveness; however, this approach does not always work where care delivery is unstructured and where scientific evidence is not available, such as in unplanned therapeutic work which occurs on acute mental health wards.

3 Gathering information through assessment is an important part of mental health nursing practice, it is an activity that is never-ending. The types of information the nurse collects should give the nurse a full picture of the service user and how they are functioning.

4 Questioning key assumptions about the nature of mental illness has led to the position that facts and values cannot always be easily separated and what appears to be a fact may indeed be a value. The uses of diagnostic criteria have changed over time (some would say they have evolved). Some might say diagnosis or applying a diagnostic label is more robust; however this process of applying a label is still dependent on the judgement of the observer.

5 This need to turn values into facts can create conflict especially if we look at the area of evidence-based practice. This approach generalises experience so a service user's self-reported behaviour becomes a diagnosis after being processed through an agreed criteria.

6 There is a need to have a shared language and using agreed terms like depression can be useful especially for research and treatment purposes, the nurse also needs to acknowledge that using the term depression provides only one version of the 'truth'. To understand a service user's experiences of their mental distress the nurse has to move beyond the use of a diagnostic term.

7 Making sense of your own values is difficult enough and trying to understand someone else's values with an eye on agreeing a way forward is a challenge. When exploring values there is a tendency to disagree as values can be quite personal, in addition when dealing with a difficult situation there is a tendency to want to determine who is right or convince the other person that your view is right.

8   It is important that the nurse respects a service user's values while at the same being clear that their actions are at times determined by codified rights and wrongs.

9   To help the nurse work through the challenges of working with values, Woodbridge and Fulford (2004) in their *Whose Values?* workbook suggest the mental health practitioner follow a good process called values-based practice.

10 Values-based practice is a good process with the aim of providing balance to the way values are manged within clinical decision-making.

6

ETHICAL RULES AND FRAMEWORKS

Background

This chapter will build on what was briefly explored in Chapter 3: the use of rules within the ethical reasoning process. To explore this use of rules, this chapter will focus on the use of legal and professional frameworks, policies and clinical guidelines all within a mental health nursing context. Ethical frameworks such as the law, the code of conduct, and practice guidelines are there to guide the nurse when making clinical decisions. Very rarely will the nurse make a decision, especially a complex one, without involving others, including the recipient of the care. Discussing these decisions with others can be useful as it assists the nurse in exploring differing options (NMC 2015a). As mentioned in Chapter 3, nurses work within and implement rules and strategies on a daily basis and of course these strategies have an element of controlling others when clinical risk is present (Alexander and Bowers 2004; Roberts 2005). The law (both statutory and common) provides guidance on what the nurse is allowed to do. In addition there is a professional expectation that the nurse will practise within legal frameworks, to 'have knowledge of and keep to the relevant laws and policies about protecting and caring for vulnerable people' (NMC 2015a: 13).

Code of conduct statements guide the nurse; however, there is level of interpretation required especially where rules appear to conflict with other rules, something we will explore further in this chapter (Smith 2012b; NMC 2015a). The nurse has to take all of this into consideration when making a clinical decision which requires an ability to reason, as well a good knowledge of the rules and knowing when they should apply these rules (Smith 2012b; Dierckx de Casterlé et al. 2008). The added pressure is that the nurse will have to do the right thing and even when the nurse believes they have done the right thing their actions are always open to external scrutiny (NMC 2015a; Mitchell 2011). If this external scrutiny happens there is the expectation that the nurse will have practised effectively:

> You assess need and deliver or advise on treatment, or give help (including preventative or rehabilitative care) without too much delay and to the best of your abilities, on the basis of the best evidence available and best practice. You communicate effectively, keeping clear and accurate records and sharing skills, knowledge and experience where appropriate. You reflect and act on any feedback you receive to improve your practice.
>
> *(NMC 2015a: 7)*

The challenge for mental health nurses is balancing the delivery of care against the need to respect autonomy while recognising that mental health care is at times inherently paternalistic (Coady 2009; NMC 2015a). There is always the question in the back of the nurse's mind; does autonomy come before the need to restrict freedom? This is a question that Michelle has to answer when working with Michael. Another question Michelle has to answer is this: at what point do I allow Michael to be autonomous? These are questions that arise from the very nature of mental health law; 'For hundreds of years, the Anglo-American legal system has been developing special rules for dealing with problems caused by the inherently perplexing phenomenon of mentally disordered behavior' (Morse 1977: 529).

Legal frameworks

Using legal rules can appear straightforward however when dealing with mental health law it is not just a case of dealing with one act:

> The Mental Health Act is one of the most complex pieces of legislation a mental health nurse is likely to encounter in practice. This complexity is further compounded by the influence of other European and national laws. In such a maelstrom of legal nuance, jargon and ethical dilemma sit some of the most vulnerable people in need of care and compassion, and the challenge of providing person-centred care in this context cannot be overestimated.
>
> *(Murphy and Wales 2013: vii)*

The legal system focuses on controlling a person's behaviour. It does acknowledge that people have free will; they also have societal responsibilities (Morse 1977). This system is shaped by the idea of 'normal' behaviour and the problems associated with normal behaviour such as crime (ibid.). To deal with behaviour that is not seen as normal behaviour, such as legal problems related to a person's mental health condition, then special rules have been created (ibid.). Historically, within the UK, society has perceived individuals with mental health needs as being more risky than 'normal' people and over recent years there has been more and more of a focus on controlling risk (Smith 2012b; Rylance and Simpson 2012). This increasing interest in controlling risk is attributed to an increase in public concern due to the media coverage of high-profile cases where members of the public have been injured and the misrepresentation of risk and it's relationship mental health problems (Walsh 2009). Due to these concerns mental health legislation has become increasingly more controlling (Coppock and Hopton 2000; Murphy and Wales).

Politics and risky behaviour is not a new issue; historically, political philosophers have directly and indirectly explored this issue from a rational person perspective. In the seventeenth century, Hobbes viewed society in its natural state as a 'state of war' and for a person to stay alive 'anything goes' that is deemed as an acceptable 'right of nature'; however, this does not include self-destructive behaviour (Pike 2000a; Hobbes 1668/1994; Wolff 2006). Locke (1679–1682) agreed that people are required to not engage in self-destructive behaviour by the 'laws of nature', they are also required to not harm others (Wolff 2006; Pike 2000b). Not engaging in risky behaviour and also having certain freedoms within a political context is based on the notion of the rational person (Wolff 2006).

A challenge with this rational person notion is that societal law is shaped by this idea of rationality and where a person is deemed not to be rational and not acting in way that meets society's requirements they can be coerced to go along with these requirements (Wolff 2006; Morse 1977). Being rational is a value judgement and by the very fact that by words and/or deeds they do not go along with the general consensus this alone could be used as an excuse for society to say this individual is not rational, if they were rational they would not disagree with the general consensus (Berlin 1998/2000). Further to this society would be within its rights to control an individual who dissents and on the basis that society was acting in the best interests of that individual and if that individual was rational they would agree (ibid.; Wolff 2006). These political decisions are based on a majority view which is viewed as being more likely right than the minority view, it can be prone to error and minority views can be oppressed and not listened to (Barry 1964/2000). In relation to mental health service users their views as a minority view are thankfully being listened too and are now having a bigger say in how mental services are being delivered which can be both positive and healthy for all concerned (Wolff 2006; Campbell 2009; Barry 1964/2000).

One real challenge for the nurse when using and understanding the law which is highlighted in the quote above is that the laws do not work in isolation they constantly interact with each and are constantly being updated (Murphy and Wales 2013). Before returning to Michael and the application of the law in this situation let us look at what is meant by the law. Murphy and Wales (2013) describe three ways law comes into being; though acts of parliament also called statue law, by secondary legislation, changes to statue law through the parliamentary process, and common law or case law where the law is further specified through court rulings. The nurse should have a good understanding of statue law and the effects it has on their practice as well an understanding of common law. In Michael's case the law allows Michelle certain powers to control Michael; however the law also ensures that Michael's rights are protected. Let us consider the main legal issues that are evident in Michael's situation.

> Michelle was aware that Michael still wanted to actively leave the ward; he also kept mentioning that he had rights. After the incident with the chair he was offered medication, which he refused, and he would not stay in a quiet space and talk, he just wanted to go home. Michael could not leave the ward as the door was locked. Increasingly he would walk to the ward door and try it to see if it was unlocked. As Michael was not willing to stay on the ward it was decided to place him under Section 5.2 of the Mental Health Act. After 72 hours this converted to a longer section (Section 2).

The Mental Health Act referred to in the scenario relates to England and Wales. Before we look at this act it is important to note that there are a number of legal frameworks that have a bearing in this situation. One such act is the Human Rights Act 1998, which came into force in the UK in 2000. This act protects the rights of the individual through a number of 'articles'. The role of the nurse is to work within these articles and ensure a service user's rights are upheld (Smith 2014). This act can conflict with mental health legislation as a service user's freedoms will be restricted where this is the case it is important that the mental health service user is informed of their rights while being detained by mental health legislation (Murphy and Wales 2013). Another act that has a bearing on the scenario is the Mental Capacity Act 2005 of England and Wales; there is similar legislation in Scotland and in Northern Ireland (Smith 2014). In this act it is presumed that a service user has the capacity to make their own decisions and; they clearly understand information relevant to the decision, they can retain, use and weigh information relevant to making a decision, and they can communicate their decision (ibid.). Where a service user lacks capacity there is a clear process articulated within the Act, this process recognises that a lack of capacity can be temporary and transient (ibid.).

The Mental Health Act (MHA) 1983 of England and Wales which was amended in 2007 provides a legal framework under which an individual meeting certain criteria can be compulsory admitted, detained and treated in hospital (ibid.). There is provision which is called a Community Treatment Order (CTO) where a service user following discharge from either a Section 3 or Section 37 can be recalled back to hospital on specific grounds (ibid.). The Act is divided into civil and forensic sections; Michael was placed on a civil section – a Section 5.2 – which is a doctor's holding power and has a duration of 72 hours (ibid.). Michael was then placed on a Section 2, which is an admission for assessment and has a duration of 28 days, two doctors make the recommendation, and the application is then made by an Approved Mental Health practitioner (AMHP) (ibid.). Scotland has similar legislation as well as Northern Ireland; the use of this legalisation is monitored by specific bodies within each country (ibid.).

Professional frameworks

In addition to using legal frameworks appropriately the mental health nurse has to understand how they fit within their professional practice, knowing the limits and boundaries of their practice (Murphy and Wales 2013; NMC 2015a). The reason this is important is that there are things legally a mental health nurse should do and things they should not. Knowing what not to do is sometimes easier than knowing what to do especially in complex situations. The NMC code of conduct advice is:

> Recognise and work within the limits of your competence. To achieve this, you must:
>
> - accurately assess signs of normal or worsening physical and mental health in the person receiving care;
> - make a timely and appropriate referral to another practitioner when it is in the best interests of the individual needing any action, care or treatment;
> - ask for help from a suitably qualified and experienced healthcare professional to carry out any action or procedure that is beyond the limits of your competence;
> - take account of your own personal safety as well as the safety of people in your care, and complete the necessary training before carrying out a new role.
>
> *(NMC 2015a: 11)*

This advice does not say what the right intervention or approach should be, what legal framework should you follow and why. This is not the function of the code as there is an expectation that the mental health nurse will know even in the most complex situations what is the right intervention or the right legal framework to adhere too (NMC 2015a; DH 2006b). The challenge for the nurse is if they do not do the right thing, work in accordance with the code, their actions may lead to a professional sanction (Coady 2009; NMC 2015a). Returning to the use of the law, the NMC (2015) code of conduct makes a number of general statements of the use of the law: 'have knowledge of and keep to the relevant laws and policies about protecting and caring for vulnerable people' (ibid.: 13), and 'keep to the laws of the country in which you are practising' (ibid.: 15).

In terms of mental health law the code makes a specific statement:

> keep to all relevant laws about mental capacity that apply in the country in which you are practising, and make sure that the rights and best interests of those who lack capacity are still at the centre of the decision-making process...
>
> *(NMC 2015a: 6)*

Again these are general statements so where does the skill and knowledge come from so the nurse can do the right thing and to know what is the right thing to do? A starting place is the mental health nurse's pre-registration training. Within this training the student nurse is expected to achieve a certain level of competency which is assessed through theoretical and practical based assessments (NMC 2010). The NMC's standards for pre-registration nursing education expect that nurses 'must be able to meet all NMC requirements when they qualify and then maintain their knowledge and skills' (ibid.: 5).

In terms of using the law there are a number of generic competencies that apply to all student nurses irrespective of their field of practice and there are field specific competencies such as the following:

> Mental health nurses must understand and apply current legislation to all service users, paying special attention to the protection of vulnerable people, including those with complex needs arising from ageing, cognitive impairment, long-term conditions and those approaching the end of life.
>
> *(NMC 2015a: 22)*

The standards then specify the types of things a first year, second year and completing student nurse should be able to do in relation to these competency statements (NMC 2010). Once registered the nurse is then expected to have the skills and knowledge to work within the code of conduct and the ability to make sense of these general statements within their practice (NMC 2015a). Even though the code has been recently changed it is still useful to consider the Nursing and Midwifery Council Professional Advisory Service (NMC 2008a) advice related to the previous code. The Nursing and Midwifery Council Professional Advisory Service (ibid.: 3–4) describes the NMC's code of professional conduct as a guide rather than a rule book, one of the reasons for this change of language from rules to a guide was to take into account how nursing practice is ever-changing and therefore it was more difficult to set rules for every situation or to be prescriptive. In the scenario where it was mentioned that the ward was locked, consider, is locking ward doors legal, and is it ethical? The NMC's (2015a) code of conduct says nothing on locking doors, although it does say a number of times about keeping people safe. Specifically, 'You make their care and safety your main concern and make sure that their dignity is preserved and their needs are recognised, assessed and responded to' (ibid.: 4).

In relation to keeping Michael safe as a good thing, it could be argued that locking a ward door keeps Michael safe, it could also be argued that locking the ward door led to Michael being frustrated and in turn led to a member of staff being injured. This could mean that the practice of door locking can be professionally a 'good and a bad thing' (Ashmore 2008; Smith and Godfrey 2002). Let us consider the law. The Mental Health Act 1983 code of practice (DH 2015a) does not say acute wards should not be locked. Instead it is suggested that:

- Locking doors should be one of a suite of approaches to manage risky behaviour.
- The negative psychological and behavioural effects of locked doors should be proactively managed.

- All service users should have regular access to outside space.
- Locking door should not be used as a replacement for adequate staffing levels.

If the nurse using locked doors does not follow this guidance on Michael's ward then their use could be potentially seen as unethical and illegal (DH 2015a; NMC 2015a).

Policies

Like the law and professional codes of conduct policies shape the way a mental health nurse practices. There are two levels in which policies do this, firstly at a strategic level and secondly at the operational level. For example a mental health ward will most likely have a policy on locking the door (see Chapter 1), however this may not always be the case or even if it is the case the policy may be difficult to find (Ashmore 2008). A study by Ashmore on locking ward doors found that nurses 'were unable to identify any mental health trust policies or guidelines available to them to support their decisions to lock the doors' (ibid.: 177).

Further to the finding above, Ashmore highlights that at the time of the study 22 per cent of wards had no policy on locking ward doors (ibid.). Operational policies do not sit in isolation they will in a lot of cases link to the law, they will also be shaped by strategic policies. For example door locking policies will link to mental health law and the human rights act, they will also talk about the need to promote recovery (ibid.). Door locking will also be linked to the way policies reflect societal trends: 'The last decade has seen an increasing focus on risk assessment, risk containment and risk minimization' (ibid.: 182).

This societal move to being more paternalistic is dualistic in the sense that at the same time there has been a greater focus on recovery (Leamy *et al.* 2011). Recovery as a term and as an aspiration is a key part of most recent mental health policies (ibid.). Slade (2012) highlights recovery as one of seven themes that occur within recent mental health policy documents:

- physical health;
- recovery;
- service experience;
- harm reduction;
- reducing; stigma; and
- well-being.

In addition mental health is now viewed in policy documents as a priority and one that should have parity with physical health (Slade 2012; DH 2015b). One such policy document according to Slade (2012) that has moved mental health into mainstream social policy is the *No Health without Mental Health* document (DH 2011). This document is guided by three general principles:

- freedom – having personal control;
- fairness – respecting equality and rights; and
- responsibility – everyone is valued.

The notion of recovery is used throughout this document which does not define recovery rather it uses the idea of clinical recovery which it suggests is just as relevant to mental health and fits with the specific use of the term recovery in the mental health field (ibid.). Clinical recovery is defined in the document as 'helping people to recover as quickly and as fully as possible from ill health or injury' (ibid.: 22). Where reference is made to the specific use of the term recovery within the mental health field the term used is based on the work of Anthony (1993):

> This term has developed a specific meaning in mental health that is not the same as, although it is related to, clinical recovery. It has been defined as: 'A deeply personal, unique process of changing one's attitudes, values, feelings, goals skills and/or roles. It is a way of living a satisfying, hopeful and contributing life, even with limitations caused by the illness. Recovery involves the development of new meaning and purpose in one's life.'
>
> *(DH 2011: 90)*

The challenge for the nurse is that in terms of both operational and strategic policy they are expected to be in control yet at the same this control has to be empowering, fair and responsible (DH 2011). How does this work in practice? Let us return to the scenario:

Michelle is committed to helping Michael to recover. She also knows that at the same time she has a duty of care to control risks, in Michael's case self-harm. Michelle has read an article by Slade (2012) during her lifelong learning journey. She decides to put what is called a four-domain approach into practice:

1   When working with Michael within the therapeutic relationship Michelle has supported Michael to identify and establish what recovery means to him. Subsequently any agreed interventions are shaped by Michael's personal definition.

2   Michelle recognises her commitment to Michael's recovery through continuing to professionally develop.

3   Michelle is working with Michael towards a planned discharge, one in which Michael can be a full member of the community and where possible engage with meaningful employment.

4   Michelle has linked Michael to service users led support groups that will help Michael to integrate back into his community while at the same helping Michael to challenge any stigma.

Michelle identified from an early stage that her practice is recovery-focused, however due to the nature of acute mental health nursing where interventions can feel almost 'invisible', not therapy but therapeutic, it was hard for Michelle to recognise how the notion of recovery fits in with her practice (Moe *et al.* 2013). During this journey of discovery Michelle recognised the difficulty of needing to be paternalistic and recovery-focused at the same time, and how local working practices and policies can exacerbate this difficulty (ibid.).

Clinical guidelines

In addition to looking at the law, professional rules, and policies Michelle will need to consider the relevant clinical guidelines or evidence-base. On this basis Michelle should be using evidence that is reliable and testable, clinical guidelines should provide Michelle with this type of evidence: 'As knowledgeable clinicians we need to be aware of NICE findings and be able to use them wisely and critically' (Newell and Gournay 2009: 4). NICE stands for the National Institute for Health and Care Excellence, an independent organisation that is:

> responsible for developing national guidance, standards and information on providing high-quality health and social care, and preventing and treating ill health. NICE guidance helps health, public health and social care professionals deliver the best possible care based on the best available evidence.
>
> *(NICE 2013: 1)*

The use of an evidence-based approach is criticised as valuing only a certain type of evidence, Newell and Gournay (2009) respond to this criticism by highlighting that 'the evidence-based movement, in general, is currently the best option we have in enriching our understanding and treatment of mental health problems' (ibid.: 4).

Newell and Gournay (ibid.) recommend that when the nurse is looking at clinical guidelines they do so with a critical eye rather than just accepting the evidence. Callaghan and Crawford (2009) recommend that the nurse develops the ability to:

* relate effectiveness, safety and acceptability to their practice;
* find relevant research;
* effectively assess the quality of the evidence;
* assess the generalisability of the evidence; and
* assess whether the evidence is applicable to their practice.

This evidence in essence relates to looking at research articles as the NICE guidelines go through a similar exercise:

> All of our guidance, quality standards and other advice products are independent and authoritative. They are all based on the best available evidence

and set out the best ways to prevent, diagnose and treat disease and ill health, promote healthy living, and care for vulnerable people.

(NICE 2013: 1)

Fundamentally Newell and Gournay (2009) focus on using evidence that is viewed as evidence-based they do not dismiss the value of other evidence such as evidence that is more naturalistic and relates to service user experiences, they just do not view it as evidence-based unless it has been through a due process.

This process ranks the evidence according to its effectiveness within clinical practice, the main research approach that is valued the most is the randomised controlled trial (RCT) and the systematic review of RCTs (Evans 2003). Evidence which is based on these approaches is the evidence that is usually used to develop clinical guidelines (ibid.).

Michelle's role is to understand these guidelines and apply them to her practice in an ethical way, considering what is the best way she can help Michael. The application of this evidence is through the therapeutic relationship. Interestingly, though a number of clinical guidelines make reference to the therapeutic relationship, there is no specific guideline. If we look at the clinical guideline for depression (NICE 2009) it mentions the importance of building a trusting relationship; however it does not make mention of the therapeutic relationship, or specifically the nurse–service user relationship. The clinical guidelines for the short-term management of violence and aggression (NICE 2015) mentions the importance of factors that underpin the therapeutic relationship and the importance of maintaining the therapeutic relationship, these are statements rather than providing detailed guidance. As the therapeutic relationship appears to inhabit the tacit realm of knowledge Michelle has to apply these guidelines in a way that fits within this realm, similar to Woodbridge and Fulford's (2004) 'two-feet' principle, values-based practice and evidenced-based practice working together.

The advantage for Michelle is that as she will have spent the most time with Michael, she should be a position where her tacit knowledge of Michael is comprehensive (Welsh and Lyons 2001; Gelder *et al.* 1983). Using this knowledge combined with using evidenced-based knowledge should enable Michelle to interpret the relevant clinical guidelines and apply them to her practice: 'The integration of clinical acumen with current best evidence will improve mental health nurses' competence and care' (Callaghan and Crawford 2009: 41).

The ability to integrate knowledge in this way is crucial, especially when you consider that a service user may have a multitude of challenges that cut across a number of clinical guidelines (Hughes *et al.* 2013). For example Michael's scenario cuts across three guidelines if we just focus on depression, violence and suicide, if Michael had a long-term physical condition such as diabetes the picture can become more complex. The challenge for any clinician whether nurse or doctor is to be able to have the time to make sense of more than one guideline especially as they will interact with each other (ibid.). One guideline may suggest one approach however another may suggest another approach that conflicts with first guideline, this is especially the case when prescribing medication (ibid.). Using a number of guidelines could lead to polypharmacy an approach which has a weak evidence-base (ibid.).

Clinical guidelines within the field of mental health nursing practice are useful however they only provide guidance which the nurse has to make sense of within their practice (NICE 2013; Hughes *et al.* 2013). In relation to Michael's situation, Michelle should access useable evidence in the following areas (Torrey *et al.* 2001; Smith 2014):

- pharmacological approaches;
- psychosocial interventions;
- wellbeing approaches; and
- self-help and psychoeducation.

Key learning points

1 Ethical frameworks such as the law, the code of conduct, and practice guidelines are there to guide the nurse when making clinical decisions.
2 Very rarely will the nurse make a decision, especially a complex one, without involving others, including the recipient of the care to be delivered. Discussing these decisions with others can be useful as it assists the nurse in exploring differing options.
3 The law (both statutory and common) provides guidance on what the nurse is allowed to do. In addition there is a professional expectation that the nurse will practise within legal frameworks. Using legal rules can appear straight-forward however when dealing with mental health law it is not just a case of dealing with one act.
4 The legal system focuses on controlling a person's behaviour, it does acknowledge that people have free will; they also have societal responsibilities. This system is shaped by the idea of 'normal' behaviour. To deal with behaviour that is not seen as normal behaviour such as legal problems related to a person's mental health condition special rules have been created.
5 Historically within the UK, society has perceived individuals with mental health needs as being more risky than a 'normal person' and over recent years there has been more and more of a focus on controlling risk.
6 In addition to using legal frameworks appropriately the mental health nurse has to understand how they fit within their professional practice, knowing the limits and boundaries of their practice. Knowing what not to do is sometimes easier than knowing what to do, especially in complex situations.
7 The challenge for the nurse is if they do not do the right thing, work in accordance with the code, their actions may lead to a professional sanction.
8 Policies also shape the way a mental health nurse practices. There are two levels in which policies do this, firstly at a strategic level and secondly at the operational level. Policies reflect societal trends such as risk assessment, risk

containment and risk minimisation. This societal move to being more patern-alistic is dualistic in the sense that at the same time there has been a greater focus on recovery.

9　In addition to looking at the law, professional rules, and policies the nurse will need to consider the relevant clinical guidelines or evidence-base.

10　It is recommended that when the nurse is looking at clinical guidelines they do so with a discerning eye, one that considers how the evidence can be inte-grated within their clinical practice.

7

ETHICAL THEORIES

Background

The aim of this chapter is to provide a brief overview of a number of major ethical theories that the nurse will find useful when ethically reasoning. These theories relate to duties, outcomes, principles and character. There is also a section on how these theories work together as a pragmatic approach to ethics. Plant and Narayanasamy (2014) highlight that nursing ethics has a long history. Its roots can be traced back to the 1870s; since that time nursing has been influenced by a number of major ethical theories, which are discussed in detail in this chapter. Over time nursing has moved into being a distinct profession with its own code of conduct. These ethical theories have underpinned the development of this code (ibid.). Ethical theories can be divided into normative and nonnormative theories.

Normative ethical theories will describe what is right and wrong, good and bad intentions, and what are good or bad character traits; normative theories can also identify ethical principles (Smith 2012b; Beauchamp and Childress 2009; Sumner 1967). Nonnormative theories are divided into descriptive ethics and metaethics, descriptive ethics focuses on the investigation of moral beliefs and conduct and meta-ethics focuses on the analysis of the meanings used within normative ethics (Beauchamp and Childress 2009; Sumner 1967). Nonnormative ethics, unlike normative ethics, is not interested in what ought to be done; it makes no recommendations. It is entirely disinterested in the moral stance a person should adopt (Sumner 1967).

Historically, normative ethics has been heavily influenced by two ethical theories: consequentialism and deontology. Over time other theories have emerged as a response to these two theories (LaFollette 2000). Consequentialism (which is also known as utilitarianism) can be sub-divided in to two prominent forms: act-utilitarianism and rule–consequentialism (ibid.). Generally, in act–utilitarianism actions are right or wrong on the basis of their actual consequences, whereas in rule–consequentialism the right or wrong of an action or act is not just dependent on the outcome, duties or rules also matter (Frey 2000; Hooker 2000). Deontology has been developed to differentiate itself from utilitarianism, as an example deontology does not hold that the right or wrong of an action is determined by the outcome of the action even if the action conforms to a set of rules (LaFollette 2000; Kamm 2000).

Out of a response to these two theories a third ethical theory emerged, which focuses on character: virtue ethics (Edwards 2009). This ethical theory is based on acquiring through learning the right character traits or virtues, the character of the person as the foundation for being ethical is associated with the writings of Aristotle (Bloch and Green 2009; Smith and Godfrey 2002). Another ethical theory which has emerged comparatively recently is principlism; this theory developed from the work of Beauchamp and Childress and has been used extensively within healthcare ethics (McCarthy 2003). Some would argue that principlism is not an ethical theory that it is an ethical framework based on a set of principles that can assist the ethical decision-making process, however due to its extensive use it is worth exploring this theory in more depth as the chapter progresses (Callahan 2003; Smith Iltis 2000).

Due to the potential limitations of using a singular ethical theory within the field of mental health nursing Roberts (2004) suggests a more unified approach is used, one that uses multiple ethical theories. A number of other authors within the field of psychiatry have also suggested taking this pragmatic approach with the view that any approach should be able to effectively deal with uniqueness of mental health practice (Radden 2004; Bloch and Green 2006). Taking a pragmatic approach means the nurse has to look at their practice first and then consider which theory or theories will assist their ethical reasoning, a bottom-up approach, rather than trying to fit a practice issue within a preferred theory, top-down approach (Cohen 2004).

Duties and outcomes

Deontology by its very name means adhering to one's duties, to not adhere to one's duties would be unethical (Plant and Narayanasamy 2014). A nurse may have a narrow view of duties especially when they think about the NMC's (2015a) code of conduct, duties in relation to deontology are wider than this, they are the duties that apply to everyone such as telling the truth, not stealing among others (Plant and Narayanasamy 2014). The NMC's (2015a) code of conduct enshrines some of these duties within a nursing context:

> You uphold the reputation of your profession at all times. You should display a personal commitment to the standards of practice and behaviour set out in the Code. You should be a model of integrity and leadership for

others to aspire to. This should lead to trust and confidence in the profession from patients, people receiving care, other healthcare professionals and the public.

(NMC 2015a: 15)

The use of the term 'personal commitment' also fits within the deontological view that doing a good act just because it makes me appear in code light does not make the act ethical (Plant and Narayanasamy 2014). For example appearing compassionate, doing the right things or going through the motions, is not necessarily ethical whereas being compassionate would be. On this basis it is not the act itself that determines whether the act is ethical rather it is both the nature of the act and the intention of the person carrying out the act that are determining factors (ibid.). Deontology is also based on the idea of reason or rational thought and that an ethical person without exception will always do their duty (LaFollette 2000; Seedhouse 2009). Reason will help a person to determine the duties to follow in a given situation:

> Our lives are governed by duties (*deon* means duty), and these can be deduced from rational principles – that is, principles any rational person would arrive at – and which will then direct our actions, if they are to be moral.
>
> *(Hughes and Common 2015: 44)*

Returning to Michael's situation, using a deontological approach creates a number of challenges. Michelle's duty would be to prevent Michael from committing suicide. Interestingly, that is also Michael's duty as a citizen. To be ethical Michelle would have to be compassionate in her approach not because the NMC says so but because it is her duty to do so. Being compassionate would be expressed through the way Michelle works with Michael; it should be authentic. Duties can conflict and in this case there is the conflict of Michelle having to respect Michael's right to self-determination while at the same time stopping Michael's determination to commit suicide. This puts Michelle in a situation where she has to choose one duty over another. Intuitively, stopping Michael committing suicide may feel ethical because Michael is deemed to be mentally unwell, not necessarily a deontological position (Bloch and Green 2009).

This conflict of duties highlights the perceived weaknesses of traditional bioethical approaches such as deontology when they are applied to mental health practice; these approaches tend to deal with the rational rather than the irrational (ibid.). In relation to deontology's respect for autonomy it is a primary duty to an adult like Michael which should be absolute; treating Michael with compassion is the categorical imperative. Considering the risk Michael poses, the problem is that Michelle also has an obligation to manage this risk and also to prevent Michael from committing suicide, overriding his autonomy, on this basis deontology does not necessarily help in resolving these conflicting obligations (ibid.).

Consequentialism sometimes called utilitarianism unlike deontology focuses on outcomes as a way of determining whether an action is ethical (Smith 2012b). The act itself is neither good or bad as a standalone act rather it is the outcome of the act that determines its ethical value, the more good the act produces the more likely it is to be ethical (Plant and Narayanasamy 2014). In utilitarianism, good can be seen in terms of 'the greatest good for the greatest number' (ibid.: 128).

Taking this into consideration the nurse has to consider carefully whether their actions produce the greatest balance of good over bad (Smith 2012b). As an example preventing Michael from committing suicide by admitting him to hospital could be seen as a good thing if it works (ibid.). If it does not work it could be seen as unethical, however the calculation of the greatest good is an aggregated calculation and you could say that most times this course of action will prevent harm and in turn be ethical (ibid.; Plant and Narayanasamy 2014). The difficulty with this approach is working out a way of accurately calculating; if a particular action led to a particular outcome, and what is the best outcome in relation to the action taken (Smith 2012b). Returning to Michael; if Michael does not commit suicide is this a direct result of being admitted to the ward and if Michael did commit suicide and it was decided not to admit Michael to the ward is this a direct result of this action? Chambers (1998) makes the point that mental health nursing is about interpersonal relationships which are complex and hard to manage, therefore a utilitarian approach may be more suitable for more simple and easily to measure interventions.

Chambers (ibid.) suggests that medical led intervention such as medication or electro-convulsive therapy may be easier to measure, however Bloch and Green (2006) dismiss this idea and make the point that it is difficult to calculate accurately the benefits and also risks associated with psychiatric treatments. The advantage of using this utilitarian approach according to Plant and Narayanasamy (2014) is that it provides focus for the nurse's decision-making activities, in essence they have to consider all options, from action to outcome, and then decide on the best course of action. Let us now return to the scenario involving Michael.

Fundamentally Michelle has to make a series of clinical decisions that focus on keeping Michael safe. These decisions are influenced by professional standards and legal guidance. Due to the generalised nature of these rules, Michelle still has to work out the detail of what she needs to do to keep Michael safe, while considering whether her proposed actions are ethical. Michelle will know her duties, she will also know she has a duty to keep Michael safe. On this basis Michelle has to control the risk that Michael may commit suicide and also take into consideration that Michael's thinking is being disrupted by a diagnosed mental disorder (in this case depression). The deciding factor or ethical justification in terms of which option Michelle chooses is dependent on the level of perceived risk Michael's mental condition and subsequent behaviour poses to himself and others. If the perceived risk is such that Michael is a clear risk to himself then Michelle has little choice but to ensure Michael is kept in hospital, not just to stop him committing suicide but also to ensure he receives treatment. Michelle will be calculating that at this juncture it is safer for Michael to be in hospital than not; he is more likely to commit suicide if he is not in hospital as he is finding it difficult to control his behaviour, which is evidenced through the assessment process. So Michelle's role is to help Michael control his behaviour in the first instance by being in control herself, and then over time she needs to work with Michael to help him control his own risk. Michelle knows that this will take place if Michael fully engages with treatment, evidenced by clinical guidelines.

Principles

Principle guides our actions as nurses both at a personal and professional level:

> The Code contains the professional standards that registered nurses and midwives must uphold. UK nurses and midwives must act in line with the Code, whether they are providing direct care to individuals, groups or communities or bringing their professional knowledge to bear on nursing and midwifery practice in other roles, such as leadership, education or research. While you can interpret the values and principles set out in the Code in a range of different practice settings, they are not negotiable or discretionary.
>
> *(NMC 2015a: 2)*

Principlism as a moral theory uses a set of principles to guide clinical decision-making, some would argue that it tries to reconcile the difference between deontology and utilitarianism (Bloch and Green 2006). By embracing key aspects of both utilitarian and deontological theories, principlism brings both a broader and more agreeable scope within the field of bioethics (Bloch and Green 2006; Evans 2000; Schmidt-Felzmann 2003). Beauchamp and Childress (2009) make the point that a key approach of principlism is not to choose one moral theory over another but to focus within a given situation on the acceptable features of a moral theory or theories. Principlism aims to provide a common sense ethical approach which is based on the rights and wrongs of human conduct (Tong 2002; Beauchamp and Childress 2009). According to Beauchamp and Childress (2009) these are widely known and are widely shared in a way they provide a stable social agreement, as a consequence a set of ethical norms or principles can be formed. Originally there were three principles which were first articulated in the Belmont Report: respect for persons, beneficence and justice. In time principlism as a moral theory has developed into articulating four principles, however these principles are similar in nature to the Belmont Report principles (Evans 2000).

Principlism focuses on the importance of these four co-equal ethical principles; autonomy, respecting and supporting autonomous decisions; beneficence, lessening or preventing harm and providing or balancing benefits; nonmaleficence, avoiding the causation of harm; and justice, fairly distributing benefit, risks and costs (Strong 2000; Beauchamp and Childress 2009; Smith Iltis 2000). These four principles are intended to be used as analytical framework within the field of bioethics providing a general framework in which more specific detail can be captured through the use of rules, obligations and rights (Beauchamp and Childress 2009). These principles are not directly mentioned in the NMC's (2015a) code of conduct, however respecting the rights of a person is mentioned throughout, as is preventing harm and managing risk, and also treating people fairly. Where principles conflict Beauchamp and Childress (2009) advocate the use of balancing; this is where reasons are identified to support a prevailing principle, and weighing which is part of balancing and this is where the relative weight or strength of a principle is considered. Taking this approach into account, Smith Iltis (2000) makes the point that it is not about finding the right answer it is about justifying the outcome of a decision in a robust way. On this basis principlism as an ethical decision-making framework is based not on the subjective viewpoint or intuition of the health professional but on a process of objective reasoning (McCarthy 2003).

Principlism can be seen as a relatively simple and transparent approach to ethical decision-making even within a mental health nursing context where paternalistic acts may occur on a regular basis (Callahan 2003; Roberts 2004). According to Edwards (2009) the key advantages of using principlism is that it is applicable to the majority of ethical challenges encountered by nurses, it provides a robust problem-solving structure, and it is compatible with the professional requirements of nursing practice.

Returning to Michael lets us consider the challenge of maintaining Michael's autonomy. Respecting a person's autonomy is an important ethical notion within everyday life as well as nursing practice; it is also one of the four principles of principlism (Roberts 2004; McCarthy 2003). Autonomy can be understood as the freedom to govern one's own life, which is free from controlling interference by others, in addition the person has the capacity for intentional action (Roberts 2004; Beauchamp and Childress 2009).

In relation to the principle of respect for autonomy, Beauchamp and Childress (2009) highlight three specific features of the autonomous person who makes a choice; they choose with intentionally, understanding, and without any controlling influences. Beauchamp and Childress (ibid.), in their preface to the sixth edition of *Principles of Biomedical Ethics*, make it quite clear in relation to the theory of principlism that autonomy is not weighted higher than the other principles. Indeed they offer a number of examples when the choices of an autonomous individual could be restricted such as if these choices endanger others or could potentially harm others, then the principle of beneficence would justifiably override the principle of autonomy (ibid.).

In Michael's case there is a need to override his autonomy due to the risk he is presenting to himself. It has to be noted at this juncture that generally it is accepted that individuals diagnosed with a mental illness may be irrational and that they can also be dangerous to either themselves and/or to others, though it also has to be noted that being irrational and/or dangerous is not necessarily connected to being diagnosed with a mental illness (Varelius 2009). On the basis of risk related to Michael's mental health condition then overriding his auto-nomy is not an uncommon practice within the fields of psychiatry and mental health nursing (Roberts 2004). To override Michael's autonomy there has to be robust justification as an outcome of the decision-making process (Smith Iltis 2000; McCarthy 2003). Edwards (2009) makes the point that where an individual is autonomous and this autonomy is overruled the burden of justification lies with those who overrule it. So where Michael is seen to have autonomy and he wants to leave the ward the nurse or psychiatrist has to justify their actions if they want to stop Michael leaving (ibid.). In addition if Michael is not seen as acting autonomously and the risk to himself is evident and the nurse did not intervene they would have to justify why they did not intervene; respect for autonomy would not be a justification for not acting in this situation (Beauchamp and Childress 2009).

Using principlism as a systematic framework for making ethical decisions there at first appears to be a conflict between the principles of respect for autonomy and beneficence, and as neither principle takes priority over the other then to find an answer the issue needs to be further analysed (Strong 2000; Beauchamp and Childress 2009). On reflection there appears to be no conflict between these principles where Michael cannot act autonomously, as this means that beneficence takes priority (Beauchamp and Childress 2009). An advantage of using principlism in this situation is that it provides a rational and calculable way of making sense of this difficult and complex ethical issue (Evans 2000). Certainly McCarthy (2003) takes the view that this systematic approach is a major advantage of using of principlism as part of the ethical decision-making process as it leads to more consistent and unified outcomes. However the theory itself does not really explain why you would follow it and as a systematic frame-work it works only where you have time to reflect on a difficult and complex set of circumstances (Seedhouse 2009; McCarthy 2006). Mental health nursing practice is dynamic and emotionally responsive. This means that ethical decision-making is not just about reason, emotions and values play a vital part and therefore it is difficult to systematise ethical judgements within this context (Roberts 2004; Thornton 2007).

Character

Character or having the right character traits is an important part of being a nurse, the NMC's (2015a) code does not mention character, however it does mention the importance of demonstrating the right behaviours:

> You uphold the reputation of your profession at all times. You should display a personal commitment to the standards of practice and behaviour set out in the Code. You should be a model of integrity and leadership for others to aspire to. This should lead to trust and confidence in the profession from patients, people receiving care, other healthcare professionals and the public.
>
> *(NMC 2015a: 15)*

It also mentions being a role model and influencing others in other words being an ethical role model (NMC 2015a). In terms of ethical theories virtue ethics highlights that having the right character traits and being an ethical role model is an important part of being an ethical person (Smith 2012b). Care ethics also highlights the importance of character traits, ones which are situated within the caring relationship (Bloch and Green 2009; Horsfield *et al.* 2011). In relation to Michael's situation this would mean that the effectiveness of Michelle's interventions are dependent on the quality of the effectiveness of the therapeutic relationship and the character traits of Michelle (Radden 2002). The types of character traits Michelle would need to possess include being trust-worthy, motivated, empathic and compassionate (Roberts 2004; McKie and Swinton 2000). It is important to note that though character and its corresponding traits are important, equally important is the application of those character traits or virtues (Radden and Sadler 2008; Smith and Godfrey 2002). As an example, being empathetic to Michael and his situation is important but it is also important that Michelle knows how to be empathetic and how to apply empathy as part of communication as a two-way process (Armstrong *et al.* 2000; Welsh and Lyons 2001; Knott 2012).

Doing good based on acquiring through learning the right traits or virtues is associated with Aristotle and the theory of virtue ethics where the character of the person is the foundation for moral agency (Bloch and Green 2009; Smith and Godfrey 2002). A challenge with using a virtue ethics approach is knowing which traits are ethical and when to use them, however the NMC's (2015a) code of conduct does provide a good level of guidance in relation to this challenge by highlighting the behaviours a nurse should possess and how they should use them. Knowing the right thing or to discern well is based on a number of factors first of all the mental health practitioner needs to possess the correct character traits or 'virtues', but also they need to be skilled in their application (Smith and Godfrey 2002). This process of possessing and also being skilled in the right character traits or virtues comes from the nurse's training, their post-qualifying practice experiences, and also their personal experiences (Radden and Sadler 2008; Welsh and Lyons 2001). This personal or you could say emotional dimension is an important part of virtue ethics. Reason and logic have their place, however they are only effective if they work in partnership with this emotional dimension (Gardiner 2003).

It could be argued that being an expert nurse is to have the right character traits and the ability to apply these traits when required, in effect an expert nurse is a virtuous nurse (Roberts 2004).

Smith and Godfrey (2002) make the point that doing good, being good, and acting on that good within nursing practice is situated within the normative practice and standards of nursing.

In addition Roberts (2004) suggests the nurse as the treater in the therapeutic relationship adopts and uses character traits which do not sit in isolation as the mental health nursing community of practice clearly identifies what character traits a mental health nurse should adopt to be an effective treater. As an example to effectively work with Michael in what is a difficult and morally complex situation, Michelle needs to be empathetic and compassionate, character traits which mental health nursing as a community of practice clearly identifies as essential traits in the relevant literature, curricula and professional standards (DH 2006a, 2006b; NMC 2010, 2015a). The practice of mental health nursing can create ethical dilemmas such as door locking which are hard to solve even if the rules are followed, however the virtuous nurse as an expert nurse knows the right thing to do (Armstrong *et al.* 2000). In doing the right thing the virtuous nurse will demonstrate, among others, virtues such as honesty, fairness and compassion, rather than vices such as being dishonest, unfair and uncompassionate (ibid.).

While doing the right thing nurses generally have to be sensitive to the individual context of care by being able to quickly respond and in the right way. It would be easy to say responding in the right way is just about logic and evidence-base but as a caring professional nurses have to also respond at an emotional level, which means that nurses have to be emotionally sensitive. The main way that nurses can be sensitive is through the use of such traits as kindness, patience, tolerance and compassion but to name a few (Armstrong 2006). In essence, an expert nurse is virtuous, and by being virtuous they become emotionally sensitive to various clinical situations in which they then have the skill to apply the right character traits (Roberts 2004; Hursthouse 1999). So being sensitive at an emotional level is not just about character traits it is also about making the right decisions (Radden 2002). Another point to note is that making the right decision generally has to be made in real time where the mental health nurse has to use practical wisdom which includes deciding what traits to use and when, they also have to be able to justify their actions (McKie and Swinton 2000).

As well as knowing the right thing to do the virtuous nurse should not be motivated by external rules they should be internally motivated to do the right thing in other words they live and in turn practice being virtuous (Armstrong *et al.* 2000). Crucial to a nurse's virtuous practice is the need to build and maintain therapeutic relationships with service users that are person-centred, empathetic and focus on working with the service user's perspective (McKie and Swinton 2000; Martinez 2009). Being expert and therefore virtuous in a real time situation is a strength of the virtue ethics approach in that it assists the nurse in dealing ethically with situational and emotional factors that cannot be predicted and only become apparent as the situation unfolds (McKie and Swinton 2000; Radden 2002). It is a flexible and person-centred approach which gives the virtuous nurse the latitude to assess and manage each situation on its individual merits (Gardiner 2003).

Being pragmatic

Using an ethical theory is dependent on its strengths and limitations especially in relation to its practical utility or pragmatism (Bloch and Green 2009; Barker 2011). A nurse may find that different ethical theories have differing utility from one situation to the next, they may also find that in some situations that a multiple theory approach is more useful. At a philosophical level pragmatism focuses on the value of reasoning as a pursuit that aims to inform practice, theorising has value but only if it is not divorced from practice (LaFollette 2000). In turn pragmatic ethics follows the same tenet in that it advocates using a multiple theory if this is the best fit for a practice situation (ibid.). Principlism has been compared to philosophical pragmatism. Unlike principlism pragmatic ethics is not based on principles but it does not mean depending on the situation that it will not utilise principles (ibid.). Beauchamp and Childress (2009) would probably view the relationship between pragmatic ethics and principlism in the same way they view moral theories in general; they do not subscribe to one specific theory rather they only subscribe to what they call the legitimate aspects of a respective moral theory. Also it is important to note that Beauchamp and Childress (ibid.) do not view principlism as a general moral theory in its own right rather a comprehensible body of virtues, principles and rules pertaining to the field of medical ethics.

Within the field of mental health, especially where service users are subjected to paternalistic acts, serious ethical issues arise which principlism may not be able to adequately address (Leung 2002; Peele and Chodoff 2009). Principlism is a reasoned approach which focuses on providing a justified and objective solution and at a first pass paternalistic acts within a mental health context can be justified especially if it is deemed that the mental health service user in question is not autonomous and is engaging in harmful acts (Smith Iltis 2000; McCarthy 2003; Roberts 2004). On further analysis the process of testing whether a mental health service user can or cannot act autonomously is not and cannot be as objective as specified by Beauchamp and Childress (2009; see also Chapter 5). This means that in relation to mental health practice principlism is not always adequate and due to its limited nature some authors such as Bloch and Green (2006) and Roberts (2004) call for an even more pragmatic approach.

Roberts (2004) highlights that only a multiple ethical theory approach can fully address any ethical issues that arise within a mental health nursing context, however Roberts only speculates what this approach would look like. It could be a mixture of ethical theories used to solve specific problems or a unified approach derived from a number of ethical theories (ibid.). Roberts (ibid.) does offer a view of which ethical theories have the most to offer, these are: principlism, ethics of care, virtue ethics and communitarianism. Radden (2004) from the field of psychiatry offers a similar view but again like Roberts does not explicitly identify what this ethical approach would look like. Usefully Bloch and Green (2006) build on Radden's work to offer a view of what a multiple ethical theory approach should look like; for Bloch and Green it should be able to deal with multifaceted ethical dilemmas inherent in mental health practice. Like Roberts (2004) this approach incorporates a number of moral theories.

The Bloch and Green (2006) justification for using this approach within a mental health care context is based on their perceived weaknesses of such ethical approaches as Kantianism, utilitarianism, principlism and virtue ethics. Bloch and Green's (ibid.) approach it is based on both a rules-based and character-based ethical approach, it attempts to address any shortcomings by using the work of the philosopher David Hume. Bloch and Green (ibid.) use Humean theory to create a balance between rule-based and character-based approaches, they determine that ethical emotions that arise in the therapeutic relationship should if required mediate any relevant ethical rules.

Obviously this approach has a medical focus rather than a nursing focus, Roberts (2004) does not go as far as Bloch and Green (2006) in the process of identifying how an ethical framework in mental health nursing would work, rather Roberts concentrates on identifying the ethical approaches which would be most useful in this framework. The starting place for Roberts is the ethical theory of principlism, Roberts (2004) takes the view that principlism is strong when ethical reasoning can be rational, universal and detached, but it is not as strong where dealing with ethical problems that are bound-up in a therapeutic relationship. To complement principlism within the context of the therapeutic relationship, Roberts (ibid.) suggests the use of the ethical theory of ethics of care. According to Roberts (ibid.) the strength of the ethics of care within mental health nursing ethics is that it stresses the importance of the therapeutic relationship within the ethical reasoning process. Roberts also sees a role for virtue ethics in terms of the impact the virtues of the nurse have upon the ethical reasoning process. Roberts then includes the ethical theory of communitarianism to extend virtues from an individualistic dimension to include a community of practice dimension (ibid.).

How would Roberts' approach work in practice? Well, Roberts (ibid.) does not give a practical example, however Bloch and Green (2006) give a flavour of how this approach might work in practice, the difference being that unlike Roberts they do not include the ethical theory of communitarianism. On this basis let us return to Michael.

The starting place for Michelle is to consider the ethical theory of principlism as a foundation for ethical reasoning. Bloch and Green (2006) suggests that principlism is useful in the process of moral deliberation in that it can complement both character traits and the care context. Using principilism Michelle reasons that she will need to be non-maleficent, avoid causing harm, the nature of what harm is will depend on Michelle's judgement. At the same time the principle of justice is important in that Michelle needs to treat Michael fairly and equally; this is where mental health law becomes relevant. At the moment this approach can appear quite clumsy especially where Michelle has to make a quick decision. Using expert judgement Michelle will consider the interplay between principlism, character traits and the care context as the conflict between respect for autonomy and beneficence becomes apparent. Michelle does not know immediately in terms of respect for autonomy, Michael's mental capacity, and on this basis it is difficult to act in this complex situation both quickly and ethically (or beneficently). By utilising the virtues of an expert (virtuous) nurse, contextualised within the therapeutic relationship, Michelle is able to be ethically sensitive and responsive to Michael's needs, allowing Michelle to quickly determine that Michael is nonautonomous and the right course of action is to be beneficent. In addition Michelle will also be able to determine what beneficent looks like for Michael; managing Michael's risk in the short-term until Michael is able to safely manage his own risk.

Bloch and Green (2006) are clear like Roberts (2004) that their ethical approach:

- utilises principles or rules;
- has to be adaptive to the uniqueness, complexity and uncertainty of mental health practice;
- is dependent on the expertise of the practitioner or treater; and
- allows responsiveness to be mediated by the quality of the therapeutic relationship.

To be an effective and ethical mental health nurses more than one ethical theory may need to be used during the ethical reasoning process. The work of Bloch and Green (2006) and Roberts (2004) will provide the nurse with a coherent way of making sense of this pragmatic approach.

Key learning points

1   Over time nursing has moved into being a distinct profession with its own code of conduct which is underpinned by a number of ethical theories.
2   Ethical theories can be divided into normative and nonnormative theories, normative ethical theories will describe what is right and wrong, good and bad intentions, and what are good or bad character traits, normative theories can also identify ethical principles.
3   Deontology means adhering to one's duties, to not adhere to one's duties would be unethical. Nursing may have a narrow view of duties especially when they think about the NMC's (2015a) code of conduct, duties in relation to deontology are wider than this, they are the duties that apply to everyone such as telling the truth, not stealing among others.
4   Consequentialism sometimes called utilitarianism unlike deontology focuses on outcomes as a way of determining whether an action is ethical. The act

itself is neither good or bad as a standalone act rather it is the outcome of the act that determines its ethical value, the more good the act produces the more likely it is to be ethical.

5   Principlism as a moral theory uses a set of principles to guide clinical decision-making, some would argue that it tries to reconcile the difference between deontology and utilitarianism. By embracing key aspects of both utilitarian and deontological theories, principlism brings both a broader and more agreeable scope within the field of bioethics.

6   Principlism focuses on the importance of four co-equal ethical principles; autonomy, respecting and supporting autonomous decisions; beneficence, lessening or preventing harm and providing or balancing benefits; nonmalef-icence, avoiding the causation of harm; and justice, fairly distributing benefit, risks and costs.

7   Character or having the right character traits is an important part of being a nurse, the NMC's (2015a) code does not mention character, it does mention the importance of demonstrating the right behaviour.

8   Doing good based on acquiring through learning the right traits or virtues is associated with Aristotle and the theory of virtue ethics where the character of the person is the foundation for moral agency.

9   Using an ethical theory is dependent on its strengths and limitations especially in relation to its practice. A nurse may find that different ethical theories have different utility from one situation to the next, they may also find that in some situations that a multiple theory approach is more useful.

10 At a philosophical level pragmatism focuses on the value of reasoning as a pursuit that aims to inform practice, theorising has value but only if it is not divorced from practice. In turn pragmatic ethics follows the same tenet in that it advocates using a multiple theory if this is the best fit for a practice situation.

8
MANAGING THE OUTCOME

Background

The aim of this chapter is to consider how the outcomes of an ethical decision can improve a nurse's future practice. During the process of implementing an agreed outcome or plan of action, the nurse will have explored different options, they will have tested the decision, and on implementation they will have reflected on their actions leading to learning which improves their future practice. Before this chapter explores this process in more detail let us return to Michelle's decision from Chapter 7.

Michelle reasoned that she will need to be nonmaleficent and avoid causing harm. The nature of what harm is will depend on Michelle's judgement. At the same time the principle of justice is important in that Michelle needs to treat Michael fairly and equally; this is where mental health law becomes relevant. At the moment this approach can appear quite clumsy especially where Michelle has to make a quick decision. Using expert judgement Michelle will consider the interplay between principlism, character traits and the care context as the conflict between respect for autonomy and beneficence becomes apparent. Michelle does not know immediately in terms of respect for autonomy Michael's mental capacity and on this basis it is difficult to act in this complex situation both quickly and ethically (or beneficently). By utilising the virtues of an expert (virtuous) nurse contextualised within the therapeutic relationship Michelle is able to be ethically sensitive responsive to Michael's needs, allowing Michelle to quickly determine that Michael is non-autonomous and the right course of action is to be beneficent. In addition Michelle will also be able to determine what beneficent looks like for Michael, managing Michael's risk in the short-term until Michael is able to safely manage his own risk.

To summarise, Michael will need to stay in hospital until it is determined that he is well enough to be discharged. The determining factor is risk; at the time Michelle is making the decision (or you could say leading on the decision), Michael has been diagnosed with 'severe' depression and he actively wants to kill himself. Of course Michelle is not making this decision in isolation; she will work within a team, and in essence this is a team decision. However Michelle is still accountable for her own practice and in this situation has to demonstrate the skills of a nursing leader (NMC 2015a). These skills or qualities include (Smith 2014):

- effective self-management;
- integrity;
- an emphasis on quality;
- motivation;
- influencing skills;
- adaptable and astute;
- change agent;
- authentic; and
- coaching skills.

In addition, making ethical decisions as a clinical leader requires Michelle to have a strong sense of moral identity which will enable Michelle to make the right (ethical) decision:

> leaders with strong moral identities are expected to reliably display ethical leadership behaviors that are consistent with their self-definitions, rather than give into pressures that would cause them to feel high levels of discomfort (e.g., unethical behaviors).
>
> *(Mayer et al. 2012: 167)*

Exploring options

Exploring all the options as a check and balance mechanism is important especially where service user's freedoms may as an outcome be restricted. The decision-making process where possible should not only be shared and agreed with the team they also need to be shared and agreed with the service user and, also the carer. In terms of decisions the NMC highlight that the nurse needs to 'encourage and empower people to share decisions about their treatment and care' (NMC 2015a: 5) and 'respect the level to which people receiving care want to be involved in decisions about their own health, wellbeing and care' (ibid.: 5). The nurse needs to encourage, empower and respect the service user throughout the decision-making process and where there is concern over the service user's capacity the nurse needs to:

Keep to all relevant laws about mental capacity that apply in the country in which you are practising, and make sure that the rights and best interests of those who lack capacity are still at the centre of the decision-making process.

(NMC 2015a: 5)

Michelle has considered this by paying careful consideration to the rules, even so there is always the concern that restricting freedoms can be inappropriate and potentially abusive (Peele and Chodoff 2009). Michael made mention to this in Chapter 4 and by expressing a real sense of frustration at the way he was being treated. Michelle ultimately felt that restricting Michael's freedoms was the right thing to do at that time; this does not mean that Michelle would have discounted completely the option to allow Michael to go home; it was not a viable option at the time.

Within this process of considering the clinical options the mental health nurse has the sanctioned power to restrict a service user's freedoms, the conditions may not allow them to use this power, however it always something that could be used (Roberts 2005). This is implicit power rather than explicit power. Explicit being the use of the power and implicit being the monitoring of the service user who is aware that if they exhibit certain behaviours explicit power may be used (ibid.). The effect of this power is that:

By creating within a client an awareness of being continually monitored … such interventions can be understood as creating and maintaining a power relation that seeks to ensure that the client regulates their own conduct in accordance with the norms promoted by psychiatry and mental health nursing.

(Roberts 2005: 36)

In other words the nurse is expecting the service user to control their behaviour, they are monitored to check whether they do, if they do not the nurse may intervene (Smith 2012b; Roberts 2005).

The challenge for the nurse is to balance this power and control against the need to be empowering and collaborative (NMC 2015a; Smith 2012b). To be balanced the nurse should not be self-serving, they have to be sensitive to do doing the right thing at the right time (Rus *et al*. 2015). Being accountable as a practitioner and a leader will provide some moderation as will the need to justify the use of power before being able to use it (NMC 2015a; Rus *et al*. 2015).

Making decisions which consider all the options is time dependent:

Identifying individual needs is the starting point for further guidance and treatment … This task is not easy. Before a solution is available, the options for care and treatment need to be explored. This exploration is a complicated, time consuming and continuously changing process.

(Wolfs et al. 2012: 46)

Where there is not a great deal of time and a decision has to be made there and then the outcome is dependent on the nurse's experience, have they been involved in a similar situation and can they use those experiences to successfully manage this new situation (Alexander and Bowers 2004; Welsh and Lyons 2001)? Berg (2008) makes the following point about experience: 'We often use the expression 'experienced clinician.' By that, we mean a colleague who is able to handle clinical situations, who is apt to judge and evaluate wisely, make good interventions and decisions' (ibid.: 152).

Turning experience into learning requires the nurse to continue to professionally develop through informal and formal learning while at the same time actively engaging in critical reflection (Welsh and Lyons 2001; Hardy *et al.* 2002). Options also have to be realistic, as an example Michelle had the option of allowing Michael to leave, however this is not realistic. It is an option to be explored but not one that is viable, Michael has been diagnosed with depression, actively wants to kill himself and if he went home it would be difficult for services to manage the risk based on Michael's history. In similar circumstance going home may be an option where robust home support is available and the service user is less of a risk, so options have to be tailored for the individual's circumstances. Exploring situations in this way requires the nurse to not only know the rules but also respond to the situation on its merits (Alexander and Bowers 2004). Sometimes to do this the nurse will feel for the solution acknowledging that knowledge is embedded within the real world and it is also embedded within the experienced nurse's relationship with the service user (Welsh and Lyons 2001; Berg 2008). Selecting the right option and doing the right thing for the service user is a challenge especially when the nurse is also concerned about not doing the wrong thing. If we return to the example of door locking on mental health wards, Ashmore (2008) makes the point that the practice of door locking is at times more about the mental health nurse covering their own back rather than being either about good practice or being of benefit to service users.

Testing the decision

This section and the next section complement each other. Testing the decision is more of a top down approach whereas acting and reflecting is more of a bottom-up approach. Both approaches relate to how evidence is collected and processed and most practitioners will use both approaches at the same time to ensure that as much evidence is collected as possible. As an example let us consider the risk management process. Nurses when making a decision about how a service user's clinical risk should be managed will base their decision on a variety of sources (Smith 2014) which will include information that is:

- unstructured and collected unsystematically such as observations of service user's behaviour;
- collected and processed through a statistically based risk assessment tool; and

- collected using specific risk assessment tools and is then compared with the nurse's knowledge of the service user and the service user's own views, this is regarded as good practice (structured risk assessment).

To use both approaches successfully the nurse has to have time to critically reflect on the evidence, this does not mean that every time a decision is to be made the nurse needs to go off and appraise the evidence (Berg 2008). On the contrary an experienced nurse who is engaging in continuing professional development should be continually appraising the relevant evidence pertinent to their practice while at the same identifying gaps in their practice knowledge they need to address (NMC 2015a).

The top-down approach is based on using the best evidence available akin to evidence-based practice; 'When EBP is delivered in a context of caring and a culture as well as an ecosystem or environment that supports it, the best clinical decisions are made that yield positive patient outcomes' (Melnyk *et al.* 2014: 5).

This process of appraising the evidence follows a seven-step process (ibid.):

- create a culture of inquiry;
- what is the question you need answering;
- search for the evidence;
- appraise the evidence;
- balance the evidence against clinical expertise and the service user's preferences;
- evaluate the outcome of using the evidence; and
- disseminate the outcome of the evaluation.

There are barriers to using this approach, including (ibid.):

- time limitations;
- lack of access to the appropriate databases and resources;
- organisational resistance to EBP; and
- lack of skill development in appraisal.

Testing a decision is also about evaluating the outcome, did your course of action work and was it the best course of action under the circumstances (Husereau *et al.* 2013). What is also important is to factor in the service user's view, not in a tokenistic way, but in a truly empowering way: 'patient empowerment has gained credibility in healthcare, reflecting moves away from paternalist models towards more equitable/collaborative models of clinician-patient interaction, including shared decision-making' (McAllister *et al.* 2012).

This approach to evaluating and testing the outcome is compatible with the values-based practice process, especially the two feet principle which supports the nurse in using a values-based approach alongside an evidence-based practice approach (Fulford 2009). Nurses will also collect evaluative evidence through the care planning process, evaluation being the stage where the nurse considers in partnership with the service user whether the plan of care actually worked (Smith 2014). Padmore and Roberts (2009) framed the evaluation stage of the care planning process as reviewing the care plan and considering the following questions:

- Were the care plan goals met?
- Did the interventions work?
- If the elements of the plan care did not work, why not, and what can be learnt?

Reviewing the plan of care or the evaluation stage should be ongoing rather than a task to be completed at the end of the implementation stage (Padmore and Roberts 2009). Where the nurse is actively engaging with the service user these encounters will be constantly providing information that can be used as part of the evaluation stage (Smith 2012a). The challenge is to make sense of this evidence, however this more naturalistic evidence gives the nurse the opportunity to explore and understand the experiences of a service user in more depth (Smith 2014). In terms of ethics this type of evidence falls within the realm of virtue ethics: 'virtue ethics resonates with my experience of life in which the nature of our character is of fundamental importance. Ethical principles that tell us what action to take do not take into account the nature of the moral agent' (Gardiner 2003: 297).

Let us return to Michael's scenario.

Michelle was sure she had done the right thing in restricting Michael's freedoms. She knew she could justify her actions. When considering the literature on depression and risk, she was provided with evidence that supported her actions. She also knew that being an ethical nurse is to be fair and honest, which means having a continuing dialogue with Michael about his plan of care and determining what Michael wants within the context of what could be realistically delivered. Michael's initial goal was to go home; another goal was not to be in such psychological distress.

Acting and reflecting

Reflection as articulated in Chapter 4 and can be reflection on action and reflection in action; these two forms of reflection are not mutually exclusive. Reflection in action, a characteristic of the expert nurse, is developed through the nurse reflecting on action through engaging in structured critical reflection:

> Reflection on action occurs after the act … while reflection in action contrastingly takes place while the situation is unfolding … However, the idea is that the practice of reflection on action fosters reflection in action …
>
> *(Amble 2012: 8)*

Chapter 4 spends some time exploring reflection on action, and Chapters 2–4, 7 and 9 spend time exploring the notion of expert practice, which is tied in with reflection in action. Taking this into consideration this section will build on the ideas in these chapters with a specific focus on reflection in action and its relationship to ethical practice. Reflection in action is a type of knowledge that is situated within a nurse's practice in addition Börjesson *et al.* make the point that:

> Schön's seminal works on reflective practice (1983, 1992) are prevailing as a way of emphasizing the value of practical knowledge and enhancing its status … Formal education and knowledge have less impact on the improvement of quality of care …
>
> *(Börjesson et al. 2015: 285)*

Reflection in action has an awareness component in that the nurse may be acting but not realising that they are reflecting, however at the moment their reflections guide their actions, such as a change in course of actions they become aware (Amble 2012). In a study by Amble it is described as 'the moment in a situation in which you 'switch on' your mentally prepared new action' (ibid.: 12–13).

How does reflection in action fit with being ethical? Crossan *et al.* (2013) highlight that self-reflection which is both reflection on action and reflection in action is an important part of the person's journey towards the developing character required to be an ethical person. As a caveat, Crossen *et al.* (ibid.) in terms of self-reflection and character trait development place more importance on reflection in action; 'reflection should be understood as reflection-in-action not simply reflection on or after action. Reflection-in-action leaves room for understanding reflection as embedded in practice and embodied in action, not simply as a cognitive function' (ibid.: 573).

By continuously reflecting on practice the nurse will not view the situation that they reflect on as separate to their development or lifelong learning journey (ibid.). The link to ethical practice occurs as the nurse starts to reason in a seamless way using ethical rules and character interchangeably. At this juncture acting and reflecting start to become one, where the nurse is starting to deal with the most complex ethical situations effectively even where a rapid response is required (Welsh and Lyons 2001). This would look something like the following:

> Schön (1983) argues that expert practitioners do not always operate on a technical rational basis. That is to say that they do not consciously call on their separate forms of knowledge, using linear, sequential thinking processes instead they respond to the feel of the whole problem…
>
> *(Welsh and Lyons 2001: 301)*

What would this look like in practice? Let us return to Michael.

Michelle recognised that Michael wanted to go home; she also recognised that he wanted to reduce his psychological distress. This was an opportunity to act and enable Michael to achieve his goals while at the same time achieving Michelle's goal of keeping Michael safe. At this juncture Michelle using virtuous character traits through the 'therapeutic use of self' started to work with Michael on self-managing his mental distress, helping Michael to understand that managing his symptoms will improve his wellbeing it will also help in the process of reducing his risk. On reflection Michelle recognised that knowing what to do was a cognitive process. In part it was also an emotional one: she could feel Michael's distress. This was important in that Michael at times had difficulty in using words to express his thoughts and feelings, and on this basis Michelle needed to know Michael in a way that went beyond words. This meant during the initial stages of their work together there were periods where there were long silences. To be skilled in using her emotions in this way Michelle used her clinical supervision sessions to move from viewing emotions as reactions to a situation to realising emotional sensitivity can help in guiding her to do the right thing.

Cultivating this emotional aspect through structured reflection is one part of the process, another part is to reflect in partnership with the service user on what lessons can be learnt from the actions undertaken (Gardiner 2003; Bowers *et al.* 2003). Listening and working with the service user's viewpoint assists the nurse not only to learn, it also helps the nurse to understand the moral and emotional tensions that can arise from a specific set of actions (Pang 1999; Martinez 2009). This process of reflecting and listening is of great value but how does this become action, and action that is ethical? Michelle knowing when to be silent and when to talk is based on the use of practical wisdom, a feature of the expert nurse (Gardiner 2003; Welsh and Lyons 2001). To use practical wisdom in a way that is seamless with the situation Michelle has to go with the flow (see Chapter 2; see also Hoff 1994; Pang 1999; Roberts 2005; Welsh and Lyons 2001). This going with the flow appears uncomplicated and simple and it will have a natural and a sensitive rhythm to the situation (Hoff 1994; Inada 1995). Going with the flow is not non-action it is where Michelle adjusts to the flow of the situation and then acts as required in a way that is not overacting (Cheng-tek Tai 2004). Flexibility is key in going with the flow but this needs to be tempered by centering where Michelle acts in a natural and spontaneous way while at the same time being wise, professional and focused (ibid.). In addition Michelle recognises that acting in this natural way, even when Michael is angry and/or stressed, will ensure that she acts ethically (Hansson *et al.* 2007; Archer 2004).

Learning and improving practice

Learning to work with the emotional dimension of practice or learning to be emotionally intelligent is a challenge (Koukkanen and Leino-Kilpi 2000; Goleman 1998). It is also part of the reflection on action and reflection in action process where the nurse through structured supervision should be supported to meet this challenge head on (Rolfe 2011). Looking at your self can be quite a difficult journey and at times quite anxiety provoking, however when working within a team it should be a process which all the team go through. Group clinical supervision is a good vehicle for this to happen (ibid.). Rolfe (ibid.) makes the suggestion that group supervision is a starting place, however to engender reflection in action it would be more useful if supervision was live. This approach involves 'a team, typically with two to four members … One member … will be actively involved with the patient, while the other team members (the supervisors) will observe and occasionally intervene' (ibid.: 174).

You could argue this happens already on mental health wards, however roles are not clearly defined and ground rules are not set. Having clearly set ground rules in relation to how teams work, especially where there is a focus on team learning promotes emotional safety (Budd 2007). By taking emotional safety into account learning as a process for change is then strengthened, as any working relationship issues that arise can be resolved through a clear and transparent mechanism which has been agreed by all team members (McLennan *et al.* 2001; Singh 2007; Budd 2007).

Let us return to Michael.

Michelle was aware that her approach with Michael was working. However, Michael still found it hard to express his feelings when talking to others, and sometimes he would become angry when frustrated. This occurred when he wanted to go for a walk and had to wait for a member of staff to escort him. At these times it was not unusual for Michael to be told that a member of staff would be available in five minutes, and inevitably he might have to wait a lot longer; sometimes his request was forgotten. Instead of reminding staff, Michael would become frustrated and then angry, and Michael would then ruminate on these angry thoughts; sometimes they would turn into thoughts of self-harm. After listening to reports at handover that Michael appeared quite angry during the morning shift, Michelle explored this concern with Michael. During this discussion, using a problem-solving approach, Michelle managed to tease out of Michael why he was angry: his escorted walk had been forgotten. Michelle explored with Michael the use of healthy coping mechanisms. Michael mentioned that going for a walk was a way of dealing with anger; it was also a way of avoiding talking about his feelings. Knowing Michael could talk about his feelings and problem solve when supported effectively, Michelle (with Michael's approval) decided to introduce other members of the team into the sessions, in order to develop a wider circle of support for Michael. Michelle also facilitated a group supervision session with a focus on looking at how staff behaviour can impact negatively on service users.

To address difficult team issues especially ones that have an ethical context, the discussion even where ground rules are present has to be collaborative, productive, and positive. Any issues that arise including resistance to change have to be overcome by the use of facilitated negotiation and agreement (Budd 2007; Hansford 2002). As an example a team can be preoccupied by saying how busy they are and that is why they act in a certain way, the trick is not to focus what has to change, but on agreeing how achieve change (Linstead *et al.* 2004).

Facilitating team change requires the facilitator to understand the importance of being emotionally intelligent in that their style of leadership has to be right for the situation it also has to emotionally sensitive to the needs of the team (Northhouse 2007; Goleman 1998; Singh 2007). Where an approach to managing change takes account of the emotional impact change then there is more likely to be a positive and productive outcome (Budd 2007; Northhouse 2007; Goleman 1998). Another potential positive outcome from this approach is that it engenders individual team members to be emotionally intelligent role models who can champion more effective ways of dealing with change (Singh 2007; Budd 2007).

By learning in this way you could argue the team is more likely to be ethical. Let us return to the individual perspective. Gardiner (2003) describes the need for the nurse with the right ethical traits to also know how to use those traits, practical wisdom which is the ability to make the right decision with the right outcome, a good choice. This use of practical wisdom described in this way can be seen to be similar to the Taoist view of 'going with the flow' (Gardiner 2003; Cheng-tek Tai 2004). Clearly being flexible and human-centred is an important aspect of expert mental health nursing practice as is the ability to be centred; analysing a situation in real time and using any arising observations to adjust practice accordingly (Welsh and Lyons 2001; Rolfe 2011). Hoff (1994) describes going with the flow, or *wu-wei*, as follows:

> You put the round peg in the round hole and the square peg in the square hole. No stress, no struggle. Egotistical Desire tries to force the round peg into the square hole and square peg into the round hole. Cleverness tries to devise craftier ways of making pegs fit where they don't belong. Knowledge tries to figure out why round pegs fit round holes, but not square holes. Wu Wei doesn't try. It doesn't think about it. It just does it. And when it does, it doesn't appear to do much of anything. But Things Get Done.
>
> *(Hoff 1994: 83)*

At times the expert mental health nurse can be seen to capture this 'simplicity' by 'responding correctly' in complex situations (Welsh and Lyons 2001). To keep cultivating this simplicity the expert mental health nurse must reflect and learn from complex situations but in a way that is not too analytical and runs the risk of losing this going with the flow aspect (Smith and Godfrey 2002; Hoff 1994). A way of doing this is for the nurse to learn from real time situations by reflecting in action and in turn develop a store of virtuous knowing (Rolfe 2011; Gardiner

2003). This store of virtuous knowledge is not just about learning rules or reducing spontaneity it is about understanding or knowing the situation and then understanding what approach did work and what approach did not work (Schön 1983; Crook 2001). Codes and rules are important but more importantly is the need for a nurse to understand the proper ethical conduct required in a real time situation (Chodoff 2009). This includes needing to know the potential harm that a particular action may cause and to understand what ethically works or does not work (Roberts 2005; Smith and Godfrey 2002; Fulford 2008).

Professionally mental health nurses are expected think or reflect on their practice especially in relation to complex situations that have a 'control' element that could lead to abuse (Welsh and Lyons 2001; NMC 2015a). Reflection is a retrospective process where knowledge and understanding are uncovered and then this process aids their future practice as stored learning (Welsh and Lyons 2001). What is also important is that this reflective process is not just a thinking exercise it also has to encompass the emotional side practice (Berg 2008). Without this feelings element the ethical nurse is engaging in an activity that is purely analytical and ceases to embed the whole meaning of the experience (Smith and Godfrey 2002).

Key learning points

1   Clinical decisions are very rarely made outside of a team. On this basis the person leading on the decision has to demonstrate the skills and qualities of a leader. It is important that in these situations the leader has a strong ethical identity.
2   A strong ethical identity enables a leader to make the right decision even in the face of strong opposition or pressure.
3   Exploring all options as a check and balance mechanism is important especially where service user's freedoms may as an outcome be restricted. The decision-making process where possible should not only be shared and agreed with the team they also need to be shared and agreed with the service user and also the carer.
4   Options also have to be realistic. Sometimes unrealistic options have to be explored; however, risk will always be a mediating factor.
5   Testing a decision is more of a top-down approach, whereas acting and reflecting is more of a bottom-up approach. Both approaches relate to how evidence is collected and processed and most practitioners will use both approaches at the same time to ensure that as much evidence is collected as possible.
6   Reviewing the plan of care or the evaluation stage should be ongoing rather than a task to be completed at the end of the implementation stage. Where the nurse is actively engaging with the service user these encounters will be constantly providing information that can be used as part of the evaluation stage, the challenge is to make sense of this evidence. In terms of ethics this type of evidence falls within the virtue ethics realm.

7 Reflection can be reflection on action and reflection in action; these two forms of reflection are not mutually exclusive. Reflection in action, a characteristic of the expert nurse, is developed through the nurse reflecting on action through engaging in structured critical reflection.

8 Reflection in action is a type of knowledge that is situated within a nurse's practice, one that appears as almost seamless. Going with the flow is not non-action it is where the nurse adjusts to the flow of the situation and then acts as required in a way that is not overacting. Flexibility is key in going with the flow but this needs to be tempered by centering where the nurse acts in a natural and spontaneous way while at the same time being wise, professional and focused.

9 Learning to work with the emotional dimension of practice or learning to be emotionally intelligent is a challenge. It is also part of the reflection on action and reflection in action process where the nurse through structured supervision should be supported to meet this challenge head on.

10 Reflection is a retrospective process where knowledge and understanding are uncovered and then this process aids their future practice as stored learning. What is also important is that this reflective process is not just a thinking exercise it also has to encompass the emotional side practice. Without this feelings element the ethical nurse is engaging in an activity that is purely analytical and ceases to embed the whole to capture the full.

9

FUTURE DEVELOPMENT

Background

This chapter will explore how the development of robust ethical reasoning skills is a crucial part of the nurse's lifelong learning journey. This builds on the ideas first articulated in Chapter 2, and developed throughout the rest of the book. As the chapter explores the notion of lifelong learning there will also be an opportunity to consider its relationship to expert practice, critical reflection and ethics as a way of life.

Mental health nurses have to manage complex clinical situations on a daily basis and in a way that acknowledges that mental health nursing as a field of practice is constantly changing (Smith 2012c). Even when challenged by constant complexity and change, the nurse will still have to deliver high-quality care (ibid.). On this basis the nurse has to possess robust clinical skills. They also have to be adaptive both in terms of their character, and also in terms of the way they deliver care (Owen and Fox 2009). Being skilled and adaptive starts with the mental health nurse's pre-qualifying training. Once the nurse qualifies they build on this pre-qualifying competency through their post-qualifying practice experiences (NMC 2010; Welsh and Lyons 2001). There is a professional commitment for mental health nurses to be lifelong learners; this commitment is now being measured through a new process called revalidation (Nishikawa 2011; NMC 2015b). Revalidation, which we will explore in more depth in the next section, is underpinned by a reflective component which require the nurse to reflect on and learn from their practice experiences (NMC 2015b; Smith and Rylance 2016). Nurses will more commonly recognise lifelong learning as continuing professional development; however lifelong learning has a much wider scope taking into account personal learning which may not relate to a nurse's practice (Smith and Rylance 2016).

Lifelong learning when underpinned by effective reflective practice assists the nurse towards improving their practice (ibid.). It is important to note that experiences are unique and dynamic and they sometimes cannot be separated from the life a nurse leads outside of their practice (ibid.). In addition both formal and informal learning should be considered equally and then reflected on in ways that both forms of learning complement each other (ibid.). Clinical supervision, (see Chapter 4) not to be confused with managerial supervision, is a common method of systematically reflecting on practice (ibid.). This method of reflection should be a formally structured activity where a clinical supervisor facilitates the supervisee to reflect on their practice with the aim of improving the care they deliver (ibid.).

Effectively engaging in the lifelong learning journey which includes reflective activities can improve the nurse's practice to the level where they are considered to be an expert (Smith 2012c). Expert nurses have expert practice skills they can also deal effectively with complex clinical situations where the outcome is uncertain (Finfgeld-Connett 2008). To do this expert nurses have to be self-aware, emotionally intelligent, they also have to be rational and logical thinkers (ibid.; Crowe and O'Malley 2006). An expert nurse uses similar skills, values and qualities to a clinical leader, which is not surprising as a clinical leader should also be an expert practitioner (Smith and Rylance 2016). To summarise, lifelong learning can lead to expert practice if underpinned by robust reflective activities. Engaging in structured reflection can also lead to being skilled in identifying and reasoning through complex ethical issues:

> Critical reflection can provide a process for identifying ethical issues and unearthing assumptions and values that may contribute to feeling 'stuck' with them, accessing other ways of seeing what is happening and finding ways to either resolve, manage, or live with conflict.
>
> *(Gardner 2014: 127)*

Lifelong learning

Lifelong learning is a commonly used concept; however, there is not an accepted definition. Koç and Erdem, after reviewing the many definitions of lifelong learning, define it as 'all types of learning opportunities that provide the individual with the opportunity to acquire learning habits and skills by means of formal or informal processes, within or outside school' (Koç and Erdem 2016: 1294).

Within a nursing context 'school' can be substituted with formal education settings, it is also a process that occurs across a person's lifespan (Smith 2012c; Tuijnman and Bostrom 2002). Common features according to Koç and Erdem (2016) include:

- Learning across the lifespan.
- Informal and formal learning.

- It benefits all in society.
- Informal learning is as important as formal learning.
- It aids skills development.
- Lifelong learning takes motivation.
- Lifelong learners are independent learners.

Within a nursing context Davis *et al.* (2014) highlight the characteristics of a life-long learner;

- They are reflective.
- They will asks questions and pursue answers.
- They enjoy learning.
- They recognise that knowledge expands and changes.
- They recognise learning as an opportunity.
- They will actively engage with learning as an opportunity.

Lifelong learning for the nurse also relates to the professional expectation that the nurse will 'keep their knowledge and skills up to date, taking part in appropriate and regular learning and professional development activities that aim to maintain and develop their competence and improve their performance' (NMC 2015a: 17). In this context lifelong learning and continuous professional development become entwined; as an added layer continuous professional development is now a component part of the revalidation process (Smith 2012c; NMC 2015b). Revalidation encompasses a number of component parts; essentially it is an overarching process that allows the nurse to maintain their registration (NMC 2015b). In addition it builds on requirements such as the standards for post-registration education and practice (PREP), the PREP standards are now part of the revalidation process, it also requires the nurse to demonstrate the continuing ability to practice safety and effectively (NMC 2008b, 2015b). The NMC (2015b: 5) highlight what is not part of the revalidation process:

- An assessment of a nurse or midwife's fitness to practise.
- A new way to raise fitness to practise concerns.
- An assessment against the requirements of a nurse's current and/or former employment.

Revalidation started in April 2016, for further information visit the NMC's website.

To renew their registration, which is every three years, the nurse will have to meet the following revalidation requirements (ibid.), providing evidence of:

- 450 practice hours.
- 35 hours of continuing professional development.
- Practice-related feedback (5 pieces).
- Reflective activity – 5 written reflective accounts and a reflective discussion.

- Good health and character through a declaration.
- A professional indemnity arrangement.
- Meeting all the requirements – confirmation.

The aim of revalidation (ibid.) is to provide a robust system of re-registration which ensures the nurse:

- Keeps their professional knowledge and skills up to date through a continuous process of learning and reflection.
- Through CPD maintains safe and effective practice and improves their practice or develops new skills where required.
- Challenges professional isolation by learning through engagement and communication with others.

Key to the success of this process is the focus on encouraging the nurse to share their learning and to reflect in a way that improves the practice they deliver (ibid.). Engaging in reflection that is robust and systematic will add value to the nurse's lifelong long learning journey enabling them to explore, appreciate, and develop their learning experiences (Smith 2012c; Eason 2010). The greatest proportion of the mental health nurse's practice is spent working with the service user, these experiences will drive the nurse's reflective activity and as they act upon those reflections the subsequent knowledge and skills they seek to improve their practice (Welsh and Lyons 2001; Finfgeld-Connett 2008). Continuing to improve practice is a component part of the nurse's transition towards expert practice (Finfgeld-Connett 2008); granted it is also a professional requirement. We will explore expert practice in more detail within the following section; at this juncture it is sufficient to mention that a nurse's post-qualifying experiences and expert practice are mutually connected (Finfgeld-Connett 2008). Benner highlights how experience and expertise connect: 'At the expert level, the performer no longer relies on an analytical principle (rule, guideline, maxim) to connect her/his under-standing of the situation to an appropriate action' (Benner 1982: 405).

In terms of ethical reasoning the revalidation process intends to strengthen this aspect of a nurse's practice by using the code of conduct (NMC 2015a) as a reference point for the requirements of revalidation, including the reflective activities that are required (NMC 2015b). Returning to the Michael scenario, if Michelle decided to used her clinical supervision reflections as part of her revalidation requirements there would be a professional expectation that she would specifically relate these reflections to the code of conduct statements; prioritise people, practise effectively, preserve safety, and promote professionalism and trust (NMC 2015a, 2015b).

Expert practice

Expert practices like lifelong learning is a commonly used term, however there is no agreed definition. Jasper makes the point that 'Although the term "expert" is used commonly in nursing practice and the nursing literature, it is apparent from this analysis and subsequent discussion that the term is ambiguous and difficult to clarify' (Jasper 1994: 775).

Taking Jasper's view into consideration there is no attempt in this chapter to define expert practice, just too merely tease out some commonly recognised characteristics. It tends to be assumed that continually working hard on a skill, deliberate practice, leads to expertise (Hambrick *et al.* 2014). This may not actually be the case. Hambrick *et al.* (ibid.), within a music context, highlight the following two myths about expert practice:

> The first myth is that people require very similar amounts of deliberate prac-
> tice to acquire expert performance ... The second myth is that it requires at
> least ten years, or 10,000 hours, of deliberate practice to reach an elite level
> of performance...
>
> *(Hambrick et al 2014: 43)*

Being an expert can be seen as more than spending time working on a skill or a set of skills, it is also about how these skills are applied, some would say that this application is the art of nursing (Finfgeld-Connett 2008). The characteristics of the art of nursing include:

- expertly adapting scientific, naturalistic, and values-based knowledge to practice;
- developing effective therapeutic relationships that meet real needs;
- dealing effectively and creatively with uncertainty;
- promoting wellbeing that is in the best interests of the service user; and
- being a lifelong learner (ibid.).

The starting place for expert practice is the nurse's pre-qualifying experiences; the student nurse's practice is developed over time through the supervisory process to be competent (Smith 2012c; Bennich 2012). Once qualified, the mental health nurse possesses a wide range of knowledge and skills. They will further refine these through their experience of being a qualified nurse (Welsh and Lyons 2001; Hardy *et al.* 2002). Moving from being a competent (novice) nurse to be an expert nurse can be seen as a staged process; these stages are described in the seminal work of Benner (1982) and include:

1 Registered nurse (novice).
2 Using practical experiences to refine knowledge and skills.
3 Competent in clinical situations, however lacks speed and flexibility.
4 Recognises and makes sense of non-standard situations.
5 Uses rules and different types of knowledge to manage all kinds of situations (expert).

The expert and the competent novice will be able to deal with a wide range of situations, however the novice will lack a degree of efficiency, and they will also not be as flexible, fluid, and analytical as the expert nurse (Lyneham *et al.* 2008; Finfgeld-Connett 2008). The benefit of being an expert nurse is that the expert is seen as being more effective than the novice especially when dealing with complex clinical situations that have no clear outcomes (Smith and Rylance 2016). This ability stems from the expert's use of different forms of knowledge: 'The expert practitioner assimilates a wide range of knowledge and understanding, which is applied to clinical practice demonstrating exemplary practical and theoretical knowledge and critical thinking skills' (Furlong and Smith 2005: 1061).

Key attributes that underpin this ability include a good level of self-awareness, being emotionally intelligent, and being committed to engage in reflective activities (Smith 2012c). It is important to recognise that these attributes complement each, reflection aids self-awareness and emotionally intelligence and to use reflection effectively a nurse needs to be self-aware and emotionally intelligent to the level that they are able to clearly identify their strengths and also their developmental needs (Smith and Rylance 2016; Arnold and Thompson 2009). This almost circular process creates knowledge which is knowledge about the self and knowledge that is embedded within the nurse's practice experiences (Smith 2012a; Smith and Rylance 2016). The expert nurse will use this knowledge not as isolated knowledge; they will use it as knowledge that anchors their scientific knowledge to their on-going practice experiences (Smith 2012a; Smith and Rylance 2016).

Being expert also means that the nurse is a clinical leader even if they do not occupy a formal leadership role (NMC 2015a; Smith 2014). Furlong and Smith (2005) highlight that expert nurses who are advance practitioners should also provide professional and clinical leadership. This leadership journey starts from the nurses prequalifying training and at the point of registration (NMC 2010) they should be able to:

- be a change agent;
- provide leadership that improves the quality of care they and others provide;
- evaluate care in a way that focuses on improved outcomes;
- be an effective time manager;
- use resources effectively;
- be self-aware;
- engage in personal and professional development;
- learn from experience;
- supervise students;
- work independently as well as in a team;
- lead the coordination and delivery of care; and
- work across professional and agency boundaries.

Returning to Michelle: as an expert and a leader Michelle recognises that she supports students through what can be quite difficult and complex situations. When reflecting on the qualities that a mentor needs to possess Michelle acknowledges that difficult situations can be ethically challenging and this has the potential to create ethical distress. So being emotionally intelligent is important, as is being honest and genuine. Michelle also has to be reliable, systematic and a good time manager, however Michelle also needs to give the student the time and space to take responsibility for their learning needs, which means on occasion being more coach than mentor.

Critical reflection

Gardner (2014) views reflection at its simplest level as 'learning from experience' (ibid.: 19). However, critical reflection is 'both a theory and a process that "involves a deeper look at the premise on which thinking, actions, and emotions are based. It is critical when connections are made between these assumptions and the social world as basis for changed action"' (ibid.: 24, quoting Fook and Gardner 2007).

Characteristics of critical reflection (Gardner 2014) include:

- having an experience to reflect upon;
- recognising the emotions and values related to that experience;
- making sense of the experience including recognising any underlying assumptions; and
- recognising the social context of that experience.

When being critically reflective it is useful for the nurse to consider the following questions (Crowe and O'Malley 2006; Smith 2012c):

- What is concerning about the experience?
- Why is the status quo being maintained?
- What are the factors that underpin and maintain the status quo?
- What is the impact upon the service user?
- Are there other options available?
- If things can be done differently what is the justification?
- Is there an evidence-base available to support doing things differently, if so, what is it?

Learning to be critically reflective starts with the nurses prequalifying training (NMC 2010) at the point of registration the mental health nurse is expected to be able to:

- learn from experience by being reflective;
- recognise and reflect on the limits of their competence and knowledge and seek advice where required;

- engage in reflection and supervision to explore the emotional impact of working in mental health and how values, beliefs and emotions impact on practice; and
- actively promote and participate in reflection which includes clinical supervision.

On qualifying the nurse, through the revalidation process, (NMC 2015b) will be required to:

- Keep their skills and knowledge up to date through a continuous process of learning and reflection.
- Reflect on the role of the Code in their practice – reflective accounts and reflective discussion.
- Compile five written reflective accounts in the three-year period since their last registration.
- Have a reflective discussion with another NMC registrant.

The professional emphasis is on the newly qualified nurse being a competent reflective practitioner who will continuously reflect throughout their professional life, in other words instilling reflection as a good habit, as a good thing to do (NMC 2015b; Smith 2012b). The challenge for the nurse is not so much developing this good habit as it is ensuring that their reflections improve their practice in a good way, which is an ethical dimension (Zande et al. 2014).

Taking this into consideration, let us return to the chapter scenario which started in Chapter 4. As we have worked through this scenario from chapter to chapter we have learnt to ethically reason using an framework with the aim of changing future practice for the better. How will this happen? Re-read the initial scenario (which is repeated below) and consider what have you learnt, what are you more aware of, and what were your underlying assumptions.

Michael is 35 years old and has recently split from his long-term partner. He has just moved back to his parents' home. He has a history of depressive episodes, which have been managed successfully with antidepressant medication. Michael has been offered talking therapies; however, he tried one session and did not go back as he did not really like talking about his feelings. This was the same picture when he agreed to go with his partner to relationship counselling – he again lasted only one session. Michael describes himself as a worrier; when asked about these worries he just says 'I worry about everything'.

A month ago Michael was interviewed by the police about constantly sending text messages to his ex-partner demanding to know if she is seeing someone else. The messages are not offensive, just repetitively asking the same question, around 100 times, day and night. His ex-partner does not want to get Michael into trouble she just wants the messages to stop; she has now changed her mobile number. A couple of weeks ago Michael was persuaded by his parents to go to hospital as he had admitted to them that while they were away at the weekend he had taken a large number of tablets with the intention of killing himself. On assessment by mental health crisis services Michael mentioned that he was worried about being seen by the police and he was having ruminating thoughts about being a bad person, he was not sleeping very well and he could not face eating food. He felt worthless, and he just wanted to die and end his suffering by any means. He felt conflicted by these thoughts and feelings as he knew his death would upset his parents, leaving him with a sense that he must get help. Michael could not give any guarantees that he would not try and kill himself again.

Subsequently Michael was admitted informally to an acute in-patient mental health ward, within 6 hours of arriving on the ward, Michael spoke to the nurse in charge and stated that he wanted to go home, his reasons were that the ward was too noisy and it was making him feel worse. After the nurse and the doctor assessed Michael he was put on a section of the Mental Health Act, at this juncture he became angry, shouting you ask me to be honest and then you treat me like a criminal. He then started to throw objects around and beating his fists against the wall, as staff tried to de-escalate the situation Michael ignored them and started to try and break the window by using a chair. He became frustrated that the window would not break so he threw the chair at a member of staff who sustained a head injury. On realising what he had done Michael stopped what he was doing sat down on the floor and started to cry, saying 'I am so sorry, I just wanted to go home to die.'

Next time you are in practice reflect on similar situations. Are you more aware of what you are doing and what you need to do? If you are, you have moved your awareness of ethical issues from being unconscious (subsidiary awareness) to being more directed (focal awareness) (Zande *et al.* 2014). In other words you are a reflexive practitioner who has become more ethically aware (Gardner 2014).

Ethics as a way of life

Emotionally intelligent expert nurses are emotionally aware of their own feelings and the feelings of others, and they are quite comfortable to work at the emotional level (Smith and Rylance 2016). They also have effective social skills which through the caring and leadership work supports them in authentically connecting with others (Smith and Rylance 2016; Settermaier and Nigam 2007). Connecting and being sensitive to others' needs in combination with being an effective ethical reasoner is an important part of being an ethical nurse (Settermaier and Nigam 2007). It is also an important part of being human, understanding your own uniqueness and being able to connect with the uniqueness of others. This includes being able to:

- understand your own cultural identity;
- appreciate other's cultural identity; and
- develop knowledge and skills that are culturally sensitive in all contexts of care delivery (ibid.).

Being sensitive to uniqueness requires and open attitude to other forms of knowledge, which can be difficult when nursing practice in the UK is dominated by a particular view of knowledge, evidence-based practice (Smith 2012a). The field of ethics is very similar, being very bioethics focused, however there is no intention on the author's part to argue we should abandon these approaches, rather we should as nurses keep an open mind (Fulford 2008). This is especially important when making sense of ethical issues within the mental health field, which requires mental health nurses to pay attention to both the evidence and the values inherent with a situation (Fulford 2009).

Opening our minds I want us briefly to consider how we can be ethically sensitive to other approaches and ideas that may be an important part of a person's identity, to be more specific I want us to be 'mindful' to other ethical values in a way that leads to being self-aware. Being self-aware is an important part of being an expert. Richards *et al.* (2010) make the point that self-awareness is a difficult concept to pin down; however it is almost certainly a psychological state where a person has knowledge of their self. Mindfulness can assist the person in developing this self-knowledge (ibid.). Mindfulness is just as difficult to pin down as self-awareness. Richards *et al.* (ibid.: 251) describe it as 'knowledge and awareness of one's experience in the present moment'. One way mindfulness assists a person to develop their self-knowledge is through mindfulness practice such as meditation or engaging in mindfulness as a therapeutic approach (ibid.). Mindfulness can and probably should be a way of life, being mindful when we breathe, walk, wash and drive; being one with the task at hand rather than focusing on future thoughts (Thich Nhat Hanh 1995). Being mindful is also part of 'letting go', a Taoist idea we explored in Chapter 2. Taoism is a name that was not 'coined' until the second century BC it relates to a number of philosophical and religious traditions that have been prominent in China and other parts of the world for over two thousand years (Eichhorn 1988; Wong 1997; Pan 2003). Of course there are a number of other Eastern philosophical traditions we could also explore; however I want to tease out other core ideas that the ethical and self-aware nurse has to be mindful of within their practice (Hawley and Lansdown 2007). These, according to Hawley and Lansdown (ibid.), include such principles as:

- Harmony – working with the whole of a person and their social networks.
- Respect – being polite, modest and compassionate.
- Hospitality – being considerate, warm, approachable and welcoming.

• Balance – being in equilibrium with all things.

Being mindful, and sensitive of another person's values takes practice and sometimes we can worry that we might not get it right even if we have a good process such as used in values-based practice (Woodbridge and Fulford 2004). Taking this into consideration, a good way to practise is to use a medium which is an important part of most people's life, yet we tend to overlook its value as learning tool: the television.

> Television has been a notorious platform for expressions that challenge social mores (e.g., interracial kisses, bisexual kisses, wardrobe malfunctions, abortion, rape, drug use and abuse, etc.). And, the increased popularity of reality television raises a host of ethical questions, not to mention a reconsideration of what constitutes 'reality'.
>
> *(Watson and Arp 2011: xii)*

Walsh (2009) offers a word of caution: 'Research carried out into the representation of mental distress suggests that mass media play an active role in the development and dissemination of a range of negative images in both news and entertainment media' (ibid.: 135). These negatives include:

• Providing one view of mental distress.
• Promoting negative and stereotypical images.
• Influencing negative images of mental distress within the public at large.
• Influencing negative images of mental distress within those who have a mental health condition.
• Influencing the government's response to mental health challenges within society.

When reflecting on a mental health issue represented within the media it is useful to reconsider the following from Chapter 4 (Shaffer and Zikmund-Fisher 2013):

• What overall message is contained within the story?
• Does the story prompt you to change your practice?
• What does the story say about how the service user was treated?
• Do you feel connected to the story, how does it make you feel?
• Is the overall tone of the story positive or negative?
• What factors could be changed to make the story feel more positive?

Try to select one issue you want to reason through. You do not always have to select the most controversial, it does not always follow that the most shocking issue engenders learning at a deeper level (Bracken and Thomas 2005). Then reason through the issue:

- What is the ethical issue, how does it make you feel?
- Identify the facts and the values inherent within the situation.
- How does the issue relate to the law, policies, and professional rules?
- Identify a relevant moral theory, does this theory help you reason through the issue?
- What is your potential solution, are there other options?
- What is your final decision, does it work, if not, why not?
- Reflect on the outcome, what have you learnt?

Key learning points

1 Mental health nurses manage complex clinical situations on a daily basis, even when challenged by constant complexity and change the nurse will still have to deliver high quality care. On this basis there is a professional commitment for mental health nurses to be lifelong learners; this commitment is now being measured through a new process called revalidation.

2 Effectively engaging in the lifelong learning journey which includes structure and reflection can improve the nurse's practice to the level where they are considered to be an expert. Expert nurses have expert practice skills; they can also deal effectively with complex clinical situations where the outcome is uncertain.

3 Lifelong learning within a nursing context relates to the professional expectation that the nurse will; 'keep their knowledge and skills up to date, taking part in appropriate and regular learning and professional development activities that aim to maintain and develop their competence and improve their performance' (NMC 2015a: 17).

4 For the nurse, lifelong learning and continuous professional development have become entwined. In addition, continuous professional development is now part of the revalidation process.

5 Lifelong learning can lead to expert practice, however expert practice is more than continually working hard on a skill, deliberate practice does not always lead to expertise.

6 The expert and the competent novice will be able to deal with a wide range of situations, however the novice will lack a degree of efficiency, and they will also not be as flexible, fluid and analytical as the expert nurse. The benefit of being an expert nurse is that the expert is seen as being more effective than the novice especially when dealing with complex clinical situations that have no clear outcomes.

7 Critical reflection is key part of becoming an expert, reflection at its simplest level is 'learning from experience'. Critical reflection requires a deeper look at an experience, one that considers the social context.

8 The professional emphasis is on the newly qualified nurse being a competent, reflective practitioner who will continuously reflect throughout their professional life. The challenge for the nurse is not so much developing this good

habit; it is ensuring that their reflections improve their practice in a good way; being ethical.

9 Expert nurses are emotionally intelligent and they are quite comfortable to work at the emotional level. They also have effective social skills which through their caring and leadership work supports them in authentically connecting with others. Connecting and being sensitive to others' needs in combination with being an effective ethical reasoner is an important part of being an ethical nurse.

10 Being mindful and sensitive of another person's values takes practice and sometimes we can worry that we might not get it right. Taking this into consideration, a good way to practice is to use a medium which is an important part of most people's lives; however, we tend to overlook the television as a valuable learning tool.

CONCLUSION

Summarising the book

This is the end of the book. However, this will not be the end of your lifelong learning journey. You may be near the end of your pre-registration training, or you may have been qualified for some time (if this is the case Chapter 9 should be useful, especially the focus on revalidation). Being newly qualified can be a stressful time; at this juncture the nurse is not fully competent and they may lack an element of self-confidence (Whitehead *et al.* 2013). It is a period of transition, being assigned a preceptor will help the nurse transition effectively (ibid.) especially if the preceptor:

- systematically supports the nurse, setting time aside for reflection;
- provides objective feedback on how the nurse's skills are developing; and
- recognises that the peer support of other newly qualified nurses is essential in the process of working through shared experiences.

Learning to be an effective ethical reasoner also takes time; similar to being supported by a preceptor it is useful to be able to identify with an ethical role model (Jordan *et al.* 2013). Good role models can also be seen to be 'authentic' leaders: 'Authentic leadership is "a pattern of transparent and ethical leader behaviour that encourages openness in sharing information needed to make decisions while accepting input from those who follow' (Laschinger *et al.* 2013: 543, quoting Avolio *et al.* 2009).

Authentic leaders as role models, according to Laschinger *et al.* (2013), demonstrate the following leadership behaviours, they:

- are open and honest, and admit their mistakes;

- support others to speak up;
- will explore difficult truths with others;
- are not afraid to show their emotions, and are emotionally intelligent;
- use their values as a nurse to make decisions;
- expect others to act on values as a nurse;
- apply high ethical standards when making clinical decisions;
- consider all options, viewpoints and information when making decisions;
- remain unbiased;
- are self-aware and open to feedback;
- have effective communication skills;
- constantly reflect; and
- encourage others to reflect and develop.

In addition the nurse has to actively engage with an ethical role model in a reflective dialogue, one that focuses on promoting learning (Gardner 2014). Through this process the nurse is creating a professional space where moral courage can be engendered, or 'commitment to stand up for/act upon one's ethical beliefs' (ibid.: 130).

I would also hope that this book engenders moral courage and in a way that supports you to clearly articulate and justify an ethical position where required. On this basis let us consider the key learning points articulated within the book. The following list provides an overall summary of those themes:

- Ethical issues are not always recognised.
- To recognise ethical issues the nurse has to be ethically sensitive at all times.
- Ethical reasoning has to be systematic and justifiable.
- Ethical theories focus on what actions are right, what ought to be done, what motives are good, and what characteristics are virtuous.
- Ethical frameworks such as the law, the code of conduct and practice guidelines are there to guide the nurse when making clinical decisions that are ethical.
- Coercion takes place through the use of implicit and explicit interventions.
- There is a strong scientific influence prevalent within contemporary mental health nursing practice.
- Mental health nurses should use tacit knowledge.
- Mental health nurses are professionally accountable for their practice decisions.
- Gathering both facts and values is an important part of the ethical reasoning process. It is important to recognise that facts may be value-based judgements.
- Truly listening to the service user's voice will give the nurse the opportunity to explore decision-making options that may be less restrictive.
- The journey towards being an ethical mental health nurse is the same journey as the one towards being an expert mental health nurse.
- Being an ethical practitioner requires the mental health nurse to possess practical wisdom, the ability to make the right choice at the right time.

- The mental health nurse needs to be emotionally responsive at all times, recognising a service user's vulnerability and how difficult it may be to make a reasoned decision.
- The mental health nurse has to manage the tension between being person-centred and empowering, and needing to managing risk.
- Professionally there is the expectation that the nurses regularly engage in reflection and this will be structured through the NMC's (2015a) code of conduct.
- Exploring all options as a check-and-balance mechanism is important especially where service user's freedoms may, as an outcome, be restricted.

Final thoughts

Refining your ethical reasoning is a lifelong pursuit, one that takes practice, patience and the willingness to seek and respond to feedback from others:

> ethical professionals do not make decisions without deliberating about sufficiently. They think through the relevant considerations carefully, gathering information as needed, and use their ethical reasoning skills to resolve ethical dilemmas effectively.
>
> *(Ford 2006: 289)*

REFERENCES

Ådnøy Eriksen, K., Arman, M., Davidson, L., Sundfør, B. and Karlsson, B. (2014) Challenges in relating to mental health professionals: Perspectives of persons with severe mental illness. *International Journal of Mental Health Nursing* 23(2): 110–117.

Alexander, J. and Bowers, L. (2004) Psychiatric ward rules: a literature review. *Journal of Psychiatric and Mental Health Nursing* 11: 623–631.

Alzheimer's Society (2014) *Dementia UK* (2nd edn). London: Alzheimer's Society.

Amble, N. (2012) Reflection in action with care workers in emotion work. *Action Research* 10(3): 260–275.

Anderson, S. (2008) Coercion. In E.N. Zalta (ed.), *The Stanford Encyclopedia of Philosophy*, http://plato.stanford.edu/archives/fall2008/entries/coercion (accessed 5th September, 2016).

Anderson, J. and Lux, W. (2005) Knowing your own strength: Accurate self-assessment as a requirement for personal autonomy. *Philosophy, Psychiatry and Psychology* 11(4): 279–294.

Antai-Otong, D. (2003) *Psychiatric Nursing: Biological and Behavioral Concepts*. London: Thomson.

Anthony, W.A. (1993) Recovery from mental illness: The guiding vision of the mental health service system in the 1990s. *Psychosocial Rehabilitation Journal* 16(4): 11–23.

Archer, M. (2004) The tao of Pooh – a philosophy that changed my practice. *British Medical Journal* 329: 151.

Armstrong, A.E. (2006) Towards a strong virtue ethics for nursing practice. *Nursing Philosophy* 7: 110–124.

Armstrong, A.E., Parsons, S. and Barker, P.J. (2000) An enquiry into moral virtues, especially compassion, in psychiatric nurses: Findings from a Delphi study. *Journal of Psychiatric and Mental Health Nursing* 7: 297–306.

Arnold, L. and Thompson, K. (2009) Learning to learn through real world inquiry in the virtual paradigm. *Journal of Learning and Teaching Research* 1: 6–33.

Ashmore, R. (2008) Nurses' accounts of locked ward doors: Ghosts of the asylum or acute care in the 21st century? *Journal of Psychiatric and Mental Health Nursing* 15: 175–185.

Avolio B.J., Walumbwa F.O. and Weber T.J. (2009) Leadership: Current theories, research, and future directions. *Annual Review of Psychology* 60: 421–449.

Bach, S. and Ellis, P. (2011) *Leadership, Management and Team Working in Nursing*. Exeter: Learning Matters.

Barker, P. (2001) The Tidal Model: developing an empowering, person centred approach to recovery within psychiatric and mental health nursing. *Journal of Psychiatric and Mental Health Nursing* 8(3): 233–240.

Barker, P. (2011) Ethics: In search of the good life. In P. Barker (ed.), *Mental Health Ethics: The Human Context*, pp. 5–30. Abingdon: Routledge.

Barry, B. (1964/2000) The public interest. In N. Warburton, J. Pike and D. Matravers (eds), *Reading Political Philosophy: Machiavelli to Mill*, pp. 224–227. Abingdon: Routledge.

Baxter, P.E. and Boblin, S.L. (2007) The moral development of baccalaureate nursing students: Understanding unethical behavior in classroom and clinical settings. *Journal of Nursing Education* 46(1): 20–27.

Beauchamp, T.L. and Childress, J.F. (2009) *Principles of Biomedical ethics* (6th edn). Oxford: Oxford University Press.

Begat, I., Ellefsen, B. and Severinsson, E. (2005) Nurses' satisfaction with their work environment and the outcomes of clinical nursing supervision on nurses' experiences of well being–a Norwegian study. *Journal of Nursing Management* 13(3): 221–230.

Benner, P. (1982) From novice to expert. *The American Journal of Nursing* 82(3): 402–407.

Benner, P. and Tanner, C. (1987) Clinical judgment: How expert nurses use intuition. *The American Journal of Nursing* 87(1): 23–31.

Bennich, M. (2012) *Kompetens och kompetensutveckling i omsorgsarbete [Competence and Competence Development in Care Work]*. Linköping: Linköping University.

Bentall, R.P. (2003) *Madness Explained: Psychosis and Human Nature*. London: Penguin.

Berg, E.M. (2008) Clinical practice: Between explicit and tacit knowledge, between dialogue and technique. *Philosophy, Psychiatry and Psychology* 15(2): 151–157.

Berlin, I. (1998/2000) Two concepts of liberty. In N. Warburton, J. Pike and D. Matravers (eds), *Reading Political Philosophy: Machiavelli to Mill*, pp. 231–237. Abingdon: Routledge.

Berlin, I. (2000) *The Power of Ideas*. H. Hardy (ed.). London: Chatto & Windus.

Berrios, G.E. (1996) *The History of Mental Symptoms: Descriptive Psychopathology since the Nineteenth Century*. Cambridge: Cambridge University.

Bertram, G. and Stickley, T. (2005) Mental health nurses, promoters of inclusion or perpetuators of exclusion. *Journal of Psychiatric and Mental Health Nursing* 12: 387–395.

Bloch, S. and Green, S.A. (2006) An ethical framework for psychiatry. *British Journal of Psychiatry* 188: 7–12.

Bloch, S. and Green, S.A. (2009) The scope of psychiatric ethics. In S. Bloch and S.A. Green (eds), *Psychiatric Ethics* (4th edn), pp. 3–8. Oxford: Oxford University Press.

Bolmsjo, I.A., Sandman, L. and Andersson, E. (2006) Everyday ethics in the care of elderly people. *Nursing Ethics* 3(3): 249–263.

Boorse, C. (1975) On the distinction between disease and illness. *Philosophy and Public Affairs* 5: 49–68.

Börjesson, U., Cedersund, E. and Bengtsson, S. (2015) Reflection in action: Implications for care work. *Reflective Practice* 16(2): 285–295.

Bowers, L. (2010) How expert nurses communicate with acutely psychotic patients. *Mental Health Practice* 13(7): 24–26.

Bowers, L., Alexander, J. and Gaskell, C. (2003) A trial of an anti-absconding intervention in acute psychiatric wards. *Journal of Psychiatric and Mental Health Nursing* 10: 410–416.

Bowers, L., Brennan, G., Flood, C., Lipang, M. and Oladapo, P. (2006) Preliminary outcomes of a trial to reduce conflict and containment on acute psychiatric wards: City nurses. *Journal of Psychiatric and Mental Health Nursing* 13: 165–172.

Bowers, L., Brennan, G., Winship, G. and Theororidou, C. (2009) *Talking with Acutely Psychotic People*. London: City University.

Bracken, P. and Thomas, P. (2005) *Postpsychiatry: Mental Health in a Postmodern World*. Oxford: Oxford University Press.

Brendel, D.H. (2006) *Healing Psychiatry: Bridging the Science/Humanism Divide*. Cambridge, MA: MIT Press.

British Medical Association (2008) *Mental Capacity Act Tool Kit*. London: British Medical Association.

Budd, F. (2007) US Air Force wingman culture: A springboard for organizational development. *Organizational Development Journal* 25(2): 17–22.

Callaghan, P. and Crawford, P. (2009) Evidence-based mental health nursing practice. In P. Callaghan, J. Playle and L. Cooper (eds), *Mental Health Nursing Skills*, pp. 33–43. Oxford: Oxford University Press.

Callahan, D. (2003) Principlism and communitarianism. *Journal of Medical Ethics* 29: 287–291.

Campbell, P. (2009) The service user/survivor movement. In J. Reynolds, R. Muston, T. Heller, J. Leach, M. McCormick, J. Wallcraft and M. Walsh (eds), *Mental Health Still Matters*, pp. 46–52. Basingstoke: Palgrave Macmillan.

Care Quality Commission (CQC) (2013) *Registration under the Health and Social Care Act 2008: Supporting Information and Guidance – Supporting Effective Clinical Supervision*. London: Care Quality Commission.

Carper, B.A. (1978) Fundamental patterns of knowing in nursing. *Advances in Nursing Science* 1(1): 13–23.

Carr, C.L. (1988) Coercion and freedom. *American Philosophical Quarterly* 25(1): 59–67.

Chambers, M. (1998) Interpersonal mental health nursing: Research issues and challenges. *Journal of Psychiatric and Mental Health Nursing* 5(3): 203–212.

Chambers, M., Gallagher, A., Borschmann, R., Gillard, S., Turner, K. and Kantaris, X. (2014) The experiences of detained mental health service users: Issues of dignity in care. *BMC Medical Ethics* 15: 50.

Cheng-tek Tai, M. (2004) Natural and unnatural: An application of taoist thought to bioethics. *Ethics and Politics* 2: 1–9.

Chodoff, P. (2009) The abuse of psychiatry. In S. Bloch and S.A. Green (eds), *Psychiatric Ethics* (4th edn), pp. 99–110. Oxford: Oxford University Press.

Chung, M.C. and Nolan, P. (1994) The influence of positivistic thought on nineteenth century asylum nursing, *Journal of Advanced Nursing* 19(2): 226–232.

Chur-Hansen, A., Taverner, R., Barrett, R.J. and Hugo, M. (2005) Mental health nurses' and psychiatrists' views on the prognosis of schizophrenia and depression: An exploratory investigation. *Journal of Psychiatric and Mental Health Nursing* 12: 607–613.

Clarke, L. (2008) The care and confinement of the mentally ill. In P. Barker (ed.), *Psychiatric and Mental Health Nursing: The Craft of Caring* (2nd edn), pp. 21–29. Boca Raton, FL: CRC Press.

Clarke, L. (2006) So what exactly is a nurse? *Journal of Psychiatric and Mental Health Nursing* 13: 388–394.

Cleary, M., Hunt, G.E., Horsfall, J. and Deacon, M. (2012) Nurse-patient interaction in acute adult inpatient mental health units: A review and synthesis of qualitative studies. *Issues in Mental Health Nursing* 33(2): 66–79.

Cleary, M., Horsfall, J., O'Hara Aarons, M. and Hunt, G.E. (2013) Mental health nurses' views of recovery within an acute setting. *International Journal of Mental Health Nursing* 22(3): 205–212.

Coady, M. (2009) The nature of professions: Implications for psychiatry. In S. Bloch and S.A. Green (eds), *Psychiatric Ethics* (4th edn), pp. 85–98. Oxford: Oxford University Press.

Cohen, S. (2004) *The Nature of Moral Reasoning: Framework and Activities of Ethical Deliberation, Argument and Decision-making.* Melbourne: Oxford University Press.

Cohen, J.S. and Erickson, J.M. (2006) Ethical dilemmas and moral distress in oncology nursing practice. *Clinical Journal of Oncology Nursing* 10(6): 775.

Commissioning Board (2012) *Compassion in Practice.* London: Department of Health and the NHS Commissioning Board.

Comrie, R.W. (2012) An analysis of undergraduate and graduate student nurses' moral sensitivity. *Nursing Ethics* 19(1): 116–127.

Coombs, T., Curtis, J. and Crookes, P. (2011) What is a comprehensive mental health nursing assessment? A review of the literature. *International Journal of Mental Health Nursing* 20(5): 364–370.

Coombs, T., Crookes, P. and Curtis, J. (2013) A comprehensive mental health nursing assessment: Variability of content in practice. *Journal of Psychiatric and Mental Health Nursing* 20(2): 150–155.

Cooper, L. (2009) Values-based mental health nursing practice. In P. Callaghan, J. Playle and L. Cooper (eds), *Mental Health Nursing Skills*, pp. 21–32. Oxford: Oxford University Press.

Coppock, V. and Hopton, J. (2000) *Critical Perspectives on Mental Health.* London: Routledge.

Crook, J.A. (2001) How do expert nurses make on-the-spot clinical decisions? A review of the literature. *Journal of Psychiatric and Mental Health Nursing* 8: 1–5.

Crossan, M., Mazutis, D. and Seijts, G. (2013) In search of virtue: The role of virtues, values and character strengths in ethical decision making. *Journal of Business Ethics* 113(4): 567–581.

Crowe, M.T. and O'Malley, J. (2006) Teaching critical reflection skills for advanced mental health nursing practice: A deconstructive–reconstructive approach. *Journal of Advanced Nursing* 56(1): 79–87

Curran, J. and Rogers, P. (2004) Acute psychiatric in-patient assessment. In M. Harrison, D. Howard and D. Mitchell (eds), *Acute Mental Health Nursing: From Acute Concerns to the Capable Practitioner*, pp. 9–28. London: Sage.

Currid, T. (2009) Experiences of stress among nurses in acute mental health settings. *Nursing Standard* 23(44): 40–46.

Cutcliffe, J.R. (1997) The nature of expert psychiatric nurse practice: A grounded theory study. *Journal of Clinical Nursing* 6: 325–332.

Davis, L., Taylor, H. and Reyes, H. (2014) Lifelong learning in nursing: A Delphi study. *Nurse Education Today* 34(3): 441–445.

Department of Health (2006a) *From Values to Action: The Chief Nursing Officer's Review of Mental Health Nursing.* London: Department of Health.

Department of Health (2006b) *Best Practice Competencies and Capabilities for Pre-registration Mental Health Nurses in England: The Chief Nursing Officer's Review of Mental Health Nursing.* London: Department of Health.

Department of Health (2010) *'Nothing Ventured Nothing Gained': Risk Guidance for People with Dementia.* London: Department of Health.

Department of Health (2011) *No Health Without Mental Health: A Cross-Government Mental Health Outcomes Strategy for People of All Ages.* London: Department of Health.

Department of Health (2015a) *Mental Health Act 1983: Code of Practice.* Norwich: The Stationary Office.

Department of Health (2015b) *2010 to 2015 Government Policy: Mental Health Service Reform.* London: Department of Health. Available at www.gov.uk/government/publications/2010-to-2015-government-policy-mental-health-service-reform/2010-to-2015-government-policy-mental-health-service-reform (accessed 5th September, 2016).

Department of Mental Health and Learning Disability (2006) *The City 128 Study of Obser-vation and Outcomes on Acute Psychiatric Wards: Report to the NHS SDO Programme.* London: City University London.

de Veer, A.J., Francke, A.L., Struijs, A. and Willems, D.L. (2013) Determinants of moral distress in daily nursing practice: a cross sectional correlational questionnaire survey. *International Journal of Nursing Studies* 50(1): 100–108.

Dierckx de Casterlé, B., Izumi, S., Godfrey, N.S. and Denhaerynck, K. (2008) Nurses' responses to ethical dilemmas in nursing practice: Meta analysis. *Journal of Advanced Nursing* 63(6): 540–549.

Dierckx de Casterlé, B., Roelens, A. and Gastmans, C. (1998) An adjusted version of Kohlberg's moral theory: Discussion of its validity for research in nursing ethics. *Journal of Advanced Nursing* 27: 829–835.

Dinç, L. and Gastmans, C. (2012) Trust and trustworthiness in nursing: An argument based literature review. *Nursing Inquiry* 19(3): 223–237.

Duncan, P. (2010) *Values, Ethics and Health Care.* London: Sage.

Dworkin, R. (1995) *Life's Dominion: An Argument about Abortion and Euthanasia.* London: HarperCollins.

Eales, S. (2009) Risk assessment and management. In P. Callaghan, J. Playle and L. Cooper (eds), *Mental Health Nursing Skills*, pp. 164–172. Oxford: Oxford University Press.

Eason, T. (2010) Lifelong learning: Fostering a culture of curiosity. *Creative Nursing* 16(4): 155–159.

Edwards, S.D. (2009) *Nursing Ethics: A Principle-Based Approach* (2nd edn): Basingstoke: Palgrave Macmillan.

Edwards, D., Burnard, P., Hannigan, B., Cooper, L., Adams, J., Juggessur, T. Fothergil, A. and Coyle, D. (2006) Clinical supervision and burnout: The influence of clinical supervision for community mental health nurses. *Journal of Clinical Nursing* 15(8): 1007–1015.

Eichhorn, E. (1988) Taoism. In R.C. Zaehner (ed.), *The Hutchinson Encyclopaedia of Living Faiths* (4th edn), pp. 374–392. Oxford: Helicon Publishing.

Evans, D. (2003) Hierarchy of evidence: A framework for ranking evidence evaluating healthcare interventions. *Journal of Clinical Nursing* 12(1): 77–84.

Evans, J.H. (2000) A sociological account of the growth of principlism. *Hastings Center Report* 30(5): 31–38.

Feely, M., Sines, D. and Long, A. (2007) Naming of depression: Nursing, social and personal descriptors. *Journal of Psychiatric and Mental Health Nursing* 14: 21–32.

Finfgeld-Connett, D. (2008) Concept synthesis of the art of nursing. *Journal of Advanced Nursing* 62(3): 381–388.

Fletcher, J.C., Miller, F.G. and Spencer, E.M. (1997) Clinical ethics: History, content, and resources. In J.C. Fletcher, P.A. Lombardo, M.F. Marshall and F.G. Miller (eds), *Introduction to Clinical Ethics* (2nd edn), pp. 3–20. Frederick, MD: University Publishing Group.

Fook, J. and Gardner, F. (2007) *Practising Critical Reflection: A Resource Handbook.* Maidenhead: Open University Press.

Ford, G.G. (2006) *Ethical Reasoning for Mental Health Professionals.* London: Sage Publications.

Foucault, M. (1961) *Madness and Civilisation: A History of Insanity in the Age of Reason* (trans. R. Howard). London: Routledge Classics.

Francis, R. (2013) *Report of the Mid Staffordshire NHS Foundation Trust Public Inquiry: Executive Summary.* London: The Stationery Office.

Franks, V. (2004) Evidence-based uncertainty in mental health nursing. *Journal of Psychiatric and Mental Health Nursing* 11: 99–105.

Freshwater, M. (2011) Clinical supervision and reflective practice. In G. Rolfe, M. Jasper and D. Freshwater (eds), *Critical Reflection in Practice: Generating Knowledge for Care* (2nd edn), pp. 100–126. Basingstoke: Palgrave Macmillan.

Frey, R.G. (2000) Act-utilitarianism. In H. LaFollette (ed.), *The Blackwell Guide to Ethical Theory*, pp. 165–182. Oxford: Blackwell Publishing.

Fulford, K.W.M. (2004) Values-based medicine: Thomas Szasz's legacy to twenty-first century psychiatry. In J.A. Schaler (ed.), *Szasz Under Fire: The Psychiatric Abolitionist Faces His Critics*, pp. 57–92. Chicago, IL: Open Court.

Fulford, K.W.M. (2008) Values-based practice: A new partner to evidence-based practice and a first for psychiatry? In A.R. Singh and S.A. Singh (eds), *Medicine, Mental Health, Science, Religion, and Well-Being*, Mens Sana Monographs (MSM) 6(1): 10–21. Mumbai: Medknow Publications..

Fulford, K.W.M. (2009) Values, science and psychiatry. In S. Bloch and S.A. Green (eds), *Psychiatric Ethics* (4th edn), pp. 61–84. Oxford: Oxford University Press.

Fulford, K.W.M., Thornton, T. and Graham, G. (2006) *Oxford Textbook of Philosophy and Psychiatry*. Oxford: Oxford University Press.

Furlong, E. and Smith, R. (2005) Advanced nursing practice: Policy, education and role development. *Journal of Clinical Nursing* 14(9): 1059–1066.

Gardiner, P. (2003) A virtue ethics approach to moral dilemmas in medicine. *Journal of Medical Ethics* 29: 297–302.

Gardner, F. (2014) *Being Critically Reflective*. Basingstoke: Palgrave Macmillan.

Gelder, M.G., Gath, G. and Mayou, R.A.M. (1983) *The Oxford Textbook of Psychiatry*. Oxford: Oxford University Press.

Gilligan, C. (1982) *In a Different Voice: Psychological Theory and Women's Development*. Cambridge, MA: Harvard University Press.

Goethals, S., De Casterlé, B.D. and Gastmans, C. (2013) Nurses' ethical reasoning in cases of physical restraint in acute elderly care: A qualitative study. *Medicine, Health Care and Philosophy* 16(4): 983–991.

Goleman, D. (1998) What makes a leader? In J. Henry (ed.), *Creative Management Development* (3rd edn), pp. 120–132. London: Sage Publications.

Gournay, K. (1995) What to do with nursing models. *Journal of Psychiatric and Mental Health Nursing* 2(5): 325–327.

Gournay, K. (2009) Psychosocial interventions. In R. Newell and K. Gournay (eds), *Mental Health Nursing: An Evidence-Based Approach* (2nd edn), pp. 95–108. London: Churchill Livingstone.

Gross, R. (2015) *Psychology: The Science of Mind and Behaviour* (7th edn). London: Hodder Education.

Hall, J.E. (2004) Restriction and control: The perceptions of mental health nurses in a UK acute inpatient setting. *Issues in Mental Health Nursing* 25: 539–552.

Hambrick, D.Z., Oswald, F.L., Altmann, E.M., Meinz, E.J., Gobet, F. and Campitelli, G. (2014) Deliberate practice: Is that all it takes to become an expert? *Intelligence* 45: 34–45.

Hamilton, B. and Roper, C. (2006) Troubling 'insight': Power and possibilities in metal health care. *Journal of Psychiatric and Mental Health Nursing* 13: 416–422.

Hansford, P. (2002) Changing Practice: Overcoming resistance in a specialist community palliative care team. *Nursing Management* 9(1): 18–21.

Hansson, M.G., Kihlbom, U., Tuvemo, T., Olsen, L.A. and Rodriguez, A. (2007) Ethics takes time, but not that long. *BMC Medical Ethics* 8(6): 1–7.

Hardy, S., Garbett, R., Titchen, A. and Manley, K. (2002) Exploring nursing expertise: Nurses talk nursing. *Nursing Inquiry* 9: 196–202.

Hawley, G. and Lansdown, G. (2007) Eastern philosophical traditions. In G. Hawley (ed.), *Ethics in Clinical Practice: An Interprofessional Approach*, pp. 101–136. London: Pearson Education.

Hobbes, T. (1668/1994) *Leviathan: With Selected Variants from the Latin Edition of 1668* (ed. E. Curley). Indianapolis, IN: Hackett Publishing Company.

Hoff, B. (1994) *The Tao of Pooh and The Te of Piglet*. London: Methuen.

Holt, J. and Convey, H. (2012) Ethical practice in nursing care. *Nursing Standard* 27(13): 51–56.

Hooker, B. (2000) Rule-consequentialism. In H. LaFollette (ed.), *The Blackwell Guide to Ethical Theory*, pp. 183–204. Oxford: Blackwell Publishing.

Horsfield, J., Cleary, M., Hunt, G.E. and Walter, G. (2011) Acute care. In P. Barker (ed.), *Mental Health Ethics: The Human Context*, pp. 197–204. London: Routledge.

Hughes, J. and Common, J. (2015) Ethical issues in caring for patients with dementia. *Nursing Standard* 29(49): 42–47.

Hughes, L.D., McMurdo, M.E. and Guthrie, B. (2013) Guidelines for people not for diseases: The challenges of applying UK clinical guidelines to people with multimorbidity. *Age and Ageing* 42(1): 62–69.

Hurley, J. (2009) A qualitative study of mental health nurse identities: Many roles, one profession. *International Journal of Mental Health Nursing* 18: 383–390.

Hurley, J. and Rankin, R. (2008) As mental health nursing roles expand, is education expanding mental health nurses? An emotionally intelligent view towards preparation for psychological therapies and relatedness. *Nursing Inquiry* 15(3): 199–205.

Hursthouse, R. (1999) *On Virtue Ethics*. Oxford: Oxford University Press.

Husereau, D., Drummond, M., Petrou, S., Carswell, C., Moher, D., Greenberg, D., Augustovski, F., Briggs, A.H., Mauskopf, J. and Loder, E. (2013) Consolidated Health Economic Evaluation Reporting Standards (CHEERS) statement. *BMC Medicine* 11: 80. Available at www.biomedcentral.com/1741-7015/11/80 (accessed 5th September, 2016).

Inada, K. (1995) A Buddhist response to the nature of human rights. *Journal of Buddhist Ethics* 2: 55–66.

Jasper, M. (1994) Expert: A discussion of the implications of the concept as used in nursing. *Journal of Advanced Nursing* 20: 769–776.

Jaspers, K. (1913/1997) *General Psychopathology* (trans. J. Hoenig and M.W. Hamilton). Baltimore, MD: Johns Hopkins University Press.

Jones, L. (1996) George III and changing views of madness. In T. Heller, J. Reynolds, R. Gomm, R. Muston and S. Pattison (eds), *Mental Health Matters*, pp. 121–131. London: Macmillan.

Jones, J. and Eales, S. (2009) Practising safe and effective observation. In P. Callaghan, J. Playle and L. Cooper (eds), *Mental Health Nursing Skills*, pp. 173–181. Oxford: Oxford University Press.

Jordan, J., Brown, M.E., Treviño, L.K. and Finkelstein, S. (2013) Someone to look up to: Executive–follower ethical reasoning and perceptions of ethical leadership. *Journal of Management* 39(3): 660–683.

Kamm, F.M. (2000) Nonconsequentialism. In H. LaFollette (ed.), *The Blackwell Guide to Ethical Theory*, pp. 205–226. Oxford: Blackwell Publishing.

Kendell, R.E. (2004) The myth of mental illness. In J.A. Schaler (ed.), *Szasz Under Fire: The Psychiatric Abolitionist Faces His Critics*, pp. 29–48. Chicago, IL: Open Court.

Knott, D. (2012) From communication skills to psychological interventions In G. Smith (ed.), *Psychological Interventions in Mental Health Nursing*, pp. 24–36. Maidenhead: Open University Press.

Koç, E.S. and Erdem, A. (2016) A comparative analysis of handling level of lifelong learning competences in social education curricula: Turkey and Ireland sample. *International Journal of Human Sciences* 13(1): 1293–1303.

Koukkanen, L. and Leino-Kilpi, H. (2000) Power and empowerment in nursing: three theoretical approaches. *Journal of Advanced Nursing* 31(1): 235–241.

LaFollette, H. (2000) Introduction. In H. LaFollette (ed.), *The Blackwell Guide to Ethical Theory*, pp. 1–12. Oxford: Blackwell Publishing.

LaFollette, H. (2007) *The Practice of Ethics*. Oxford: Blackwell Publishing.

Lamza, C. and Smith, P. (2014) Values-based training for mental health nurses. *Nursing Times* 110(15): 22–24.

Lane, D.A. and Corrie, S. (2012) *Making Successful Decisions in Counselling and Psychotherapy: A Practical Guide*. Maidenhead: McGraw Hill.

Laschinger, H.K.S., Wong, C.A. and Grau, A.L. (2013) Authentic leadership, empowerment and burnout: a comparison in new graduates and experienced nurses. *Journal of Nursing Management* 21(3): 541–552.

Leamy, M., Bird, V., Le Boutillier, C., Williams, J. and Slade, M. (2011) Conceptual framework for personal recovery in mental health: systematic review and narrative synthesis. *The British Journal of Psychiatry* 199(6): 445–452.

Leff, J. (2001) *The Unbalanced Mind*. London: Weidenfeld & Nicolson.

Leung, W. (2002) Why the professional–client ethic is inadequate in mental health care. *Nursing Ethics* 9(1): 51–60.

Liégeois, A. and Eneman, M. (2008) Ethics of deliberation, consent and coercion in psychiatry. *Journal of Medical Ethics* 34: 73–76.

Linstead, S., Fulop, L. and Lilley, S. (2004) *Management and Organisation: A Critical Text*. Basingstoke: Palgrave Macmillan.

Lyneham, J., Parkinson, C. and Denholm, C. (2008) Explicating Benner's concept of expert practice: intuition in emergency nursing. *Journal of Advanced Nursing* 64(4): 380–387.

Martinez, R. (2009) Narrative ethics. In S. Bloch and S.A. Green (eds), *Psychiatric Ethics* (4th edn), pp. 49–60. Oxford: Oxford University Press.

Mayer, D.M., Aquino, K., Greenbaum, R.L. and Kuenzi, M. (2012) Who displays ethical leadership, and why does it matter? An examination of antecedents and consequences of ethical leadership. *Academy of Management Journal* 55(1): 151–171.

McAllister, M., Dunn, G., Payne, K., Davies, L. and Todd, C. (2012) Patient empowerment: The need to consider it as a measurable patient-reported outcome for chronic conditions. *BMC Health Services Research* 12(1): 157.

McAndrew, S., Chambers, M., Nolan, F., Thomas, B. and Watts, P. (2014) Measuring the evidence: Reviewing the literature of the measurement of therapeutic engagement in acute mental health inpatient wards. *International Journal of Mental Health Nursing* 23(3): 212–220.

McCarthy, J. (2003) Principlism or narrative ethics: Must we choose between them? *Medical Humanities* 29: 65–71.

McCarthy, J. (2006) A pluralist view of nursing ethics. *Nursing Philosophy* 7: 157–164.

McKie, A. and Swinton, J. (2000) Community, culture and character: The place of virtues in psychiatric nursing practice. *Journal of Psychiatric and Mental Health Nursing* 7: 35–42.

McLennan, A., Banks, D., Gass, J., Gault. B. and McKie, A. (2001) Similarities not differences: An exploration of the impact of change upon a group of nursing lecturers within a university setting. *Nurse Education Today* 21(5): 391–397.

Melnyk, B.M., Gallagher Ford, L., Long, L.E. and Fineout Overholt, E. (2014) The establishment of evidence based practice competencies for practicing registered nurses and advanced practice nurses in real world clinical settings: Proficiencies to improve healthcare quality, reliability, patient outcomes, and costs. *Worldviews on Evidence Based Nursing* 11(1): 5–15.

Mental Capacity Implementation Programme (2009) *Making Decisions … About Your Health, Welfare or Finances: Who Decides When You Can't?* (4th edn). London: The Mental Capacity Implementation Programme.

Mental Health Foundation (2009) *Model Values? Race, Values and Models in Mental Health.* London: Mental Health Foundation.

Merleau-Ponty, M. (1945/1962) *The Phenomenology of Perception* (trans. C. Smith). London: Routledge.

Mitchell, V. (2011) Professional relationships. In P. Barker (ed.), *Mental Health Ethics: The Human Context*, pp. 149–158. London: Routledge.

Moe, C., Kvig, E.I., Brinchmann, B. and Brinchmann, B.S. (2013) Working behind the scenes: An ethical view of mental health nursing and first-episode psychosis. *Nursing Ethics* 20(5): 517–527.

Morgan, A., Felton, A., Fulford, K.W.M., Kalathil, J. and Stacey, G. (2016) *Values and Ethics in Mental Health: An Exploration for Practice*. London: Palgrave Macmillan.

Morrison, J. (2014) *Diagnosis Made Easier: Principles and Techniques for Mental Health Clinicians.* New York: Guildford Press.

Morrison, S.M. and Symes, L. (2011) An integrative review of expert nursing practice. *Journal of Nursing Scholarship* 43(2): 163–170.

Morse, S.J. (1977) Crazy behavior, morals, and science: An analysis of mental health law. *Southern California Law Review* 51: 527–654.

Murphy, R. and Wales, P. (2013) *Mental Health Law in Nursing*. London: Learning Matters.

New Scientist (1997) Editorial: Inadmissible evidence. *New Scientist* (22 March): 3.

Newell, R. and Gournay, K. (2009) Introduction: Evidence in mental health care. In R. Newell and K. Gournay (eds), *Mental Health Nursing: An Evidence-Based Approach* (2nd edn), pp. 1–6. London: Churchill Livingstone.

NICE (2009) *Depression in Adults: Recognition and Management*. Clinical Guideline 90. London: National Institute for Health and Clinical Excellence.

NICE (2013) *NICE Charter*. London: National Institute for Health and Clinical Excellence.

NICE (2015) *Violence and Aggression: Short-Term Management in Mental Health, Health and Community Settings*. Clinical Guideline 39. London: National Institute for Health and Clinical Excellence.

Nishikawa, M. (2011) (Re)defining care workers as knowledge workers. *Gender, Work and Organization* 18: 113–136.

Nolan, P. (1993) *A History of Mental Health Nursing*. Cheltenham: Stanley Thornes.

Northhouse, P.G. (2007) *Leadership: Theory and Practice* (4th edn). London: Sage Publications.

Nursing & Midwifery Council (2006) *A–Z Advice Sheet C: Clinical Supervision*. London: NMC.

Nursing & Midwifery Council (2008a) The Code: Standards of conduct, performance and ethics for nurses and midwives. *Nursing Times* 104(17): 1–16.

Nursing & Midwifery Council (2008b) *The Prep Handbook*. London: Nursing and Midwifery Council.

Nursing & Midwifery Council (2010) *Standards for Pre-registration Nursing Education*. London: Nursing and Midwifery Council.

Nursing & Midwifery Council (2015a) *The Code: Professional Standards of Practice and Behaviour for Nurses and Midwives*. London: Nursing and Midwifery Council.

Nursing & Midwifery Council (2015b) *Revalidation: How to Revalidate with the NMC – Requirements for Renewing your Registration*. London: Nursing and Midwifery Council.

O'Brien, A.J. and Golding, C.G. (2003) Coercion in mental healthcare: The principle of least coercive care. *Journal of Psychiatric and Mental Health Nursing* 10: 167–173.

Owen, S. and Fox, C. (2009) Personal and professional development. In P. Callaghan, J. Playle and L. Cooper (eds), *Mental Health Nursing Skills*, pp. 223–231. Oxford: Oxford University Press.

Oyebode, F. (2008) *Sims' Symptoms in the Mind: An Introduction to Descriptive Psychopathology* (4th edn). London: Saunders.

Padmore, J. and Roberts, C. (2009) Care planning. In I. Norman and I. Ryrie (eds), *The Art and Science of Mental Health Nursing: Principles and Practice* (3rd edn), pp. 221–232. Maidenhead: Open University Press.

Pan, D. (2003) The Tao of a peaceful mind: the representation of emotional health and healing in traditional Chinese literature. *Mental Health, Religion and Culture* 6(3): 241–259.

Pang, M.S. (1999) Protective truthfulness: the Chinese way of safeguarding patients in informed treatment decisions. *Journal of Medical Ethics* 25: 247–253.

Peele, R. and Chodoff, P. (2009) Involuntary hospitalization and deinstitutionalization. In S. Bloch and S.A. Green (eds), *Psychiatric Ethics* (4th edn), pp. 211–228. Oxford: Oxford University Press.

Perraud, S., Delaney, K.R., Carlson-Sabelli, L., Johnson, M.E., Shephard, R. and Paun, O. (2006) Advanced practice psychiatric mental health nursing, finding our core: The therapeutic relationship in 21st century, *Perspectives in Psychiatric Care* 42(4): 215–226.

Pike, J. (2000a) Thomas Hobbes: Leviathan. In N. Warburton, J. Pike and D. Matravers (eds), *Reading Political Philosophy: Machiavelli to Mill*, pp. 68–134. Abingdon: Routledge.

Pike, J. (2000b) John Locke: The Second Treatise of Government. In N. Warburton, J. Pike and D. Matravers (eds), *Reading Political Philosophy: Machiavelli to Mill*, pp. 135–184. Abingdon: Routledge.

Plant, N. and Narayanasamy, A. (2014) Ethical theories. In T. Stickley, and N. Wright (eds), *Mental Health Nursing: A Guide for Practice*, pp. 122–133. London: Sage.

Polanyi, M. (1958) *Personal Knowledge: Towards a Post-Critical Philosophy*. Chicago, IL: University of Chicago Press.

Porter, R. (2002) *Madness: A Brief History*. Oxford: Oxford University Press.

Radden, J. (2002) Notes towards a professional ethics for psychiatry. *Australian and New Zealand Journal of Psychiatry* 36: 52–59.

Radden, J. (2004) The nature and scope of psychiatric ethics. *South African Psychiatry Review* 7: 4–9.

Radden, J. and Sadler, J.Z. (2008) Character virtues in psychiatric practice. *Harvard Review of Psychiatry* 16(6): 373–380.

Read, J. (2004) A history of madness. In J. Read, L.R. Mosher and R.P. Bentall (eds), *Models of Madness*, pp. 9–20. London: Routledge.

Redfield Jamison, K. (2000) *Night Falls Fast: Understanding Suicide*. London: Picador.

Rest, J.R. (1986) *Moral Development: Advances in Research and Theory*. New York: Praeger.

Reynolds, B. (2008) Developing empathy. In P. Barker (ed.), *Psychiatric and Mental Health Nursing: The Craft of Caring* (2nd edn), pp. 321–329. Boca Raton, FL: CRC Press.

Rhodes, R. and Alfandre, D. (2007) A systematic approach to clinical moral reasoning. *Clinical Ethics* 2: 66–70.

Richards, K.C., Campenni, C.E. and Muse-Burke, J.L. (2010) Self-care and well-being in mental health professionals: The mediating effects of self-awareness and mindfulness. *Journal of Mental Health Counseling* 32(3): 247.

Ripstein, A. (2004) Authority and coercion. *Philosophy and Public Affairs* 33(1): 2–35.

Roberts, M. (2004) Psychiatric ethics: A critical introduction for mental health nurses. *Journal of Psychiatric and Mental Health Nursing* 11: 583–588.

Roberts, M. (2005) The production of the psychiatric subject: Power, knowledge and Michel Foucault. *Nursing Philosophy* 6: 33–42.

Rolfe, G. (2011) Reflection-in-action. In G. Rolfe, M. Jasper and D. Freshwater (eds), *Critical Reflection in Practice: Generating Knowledge for Care* (2nd edn), pp. 160–182. Basingstoke: Palgrave Macmillan.

Rus, D., van Knippenberg, D. and Wisse, B. (2012) Leader power and self-serving behavior: The moderating role of accountability. *The Leadership Quarterly* 23(1): 13–26.

Rylance, R. and Simpson, P. (2012) Psychological interventions and managing risk. In G. Smith (ed.), *Psychological Interventions in Mental Health Nursing*, pp. 11–23. Maidenhead: Open University Press.

Schmidt-Felzmann, H. (2003) Pragmatic principles: Methodological pragmatism in the principle-based approach to bioethics. *Journal of Medicine and Philosophy* 28(5/6): 581–596.

Schön, D. (1983) *The Reflective Practitioner: How Professionals Think in Action*. New York: Basic Books.

Schön, D. (1992) The theory of inquiry: Dewey's legacy to education. *Curriculum Inquiry* 22: 119–139.

Scottish Executive (2006) *Rights, Relationships, and Recovery: The Report of the National Review of Mental Health Nursing in Scotland*. Edinburgh: Scottish Executive.

Seedhouse, D. (2009) *Ethics: The Heart of Health Care* (3rd edn). Chichester: John Wiley & Sons.

Settermaier, E. and Nigam, M. (2007) Where did you get your values and beliefs? In G. Hawley (ed.), *Ethics in Clinical Practice: An Interprofessional Approach*, pp. 15–34. London: Pearson Education.

Shaffer, V.A. and Zikmund-Fisher, B.J. (2013) All stories are not alike: A purpose-, content-, and valence-based taxonomy of patient narratives in decision aids. *Medical Decision Making* 33: 4–13.

Shipley, S.D. (2010) Listening: A concept analysis. *Nursing Forum* 45(2): 125–134.

Shorter, E. (1997) *A History of Psychiatry: From the Era of the Asylum to the Age of Prozac*. New York: John Wiley & Sons.

Silverstein, C.M. (2006) Therapeutic interpersonal interactions: The sacrificial lamb? *Perspectives in Psychiatric Care* 42(1): 33–41.

Sims, A.C.P. (2003) *Symptoms in the Mind: An Introduction to Descriptive Psychopathology*. London: Saunders.

Singh, S.K. (2007) Role of emotional intelligence in organisational learning: An empirical study. *Singapore Management Review* 29(2): 55–74.

Slade, M. (2012) Everyday solutions for everyday problems: How mental health systems can support recovery. *Psychiatric Services* 63(7): 702–704.

Smith, G. (2012a) An introduction to psychological interventions. In G. Smith (ed.), *Psychological Interventions in Mental Health Nursing*, pp. 1–10. Maidenhead: Open University Press.

Smith, G. (2012b) Psychological interventions within an ethical context. In G. Smith (ed.), *Psychological Interventions in Mental Health Nursing*, pp. 143–154. Maidenhead: Open University Press.

Smith, G. (2012c) Conclusion: Psychological interventions and the mental health nurse's future development. In G. Smith (ed.), *Psychological Interventions in Mental Health Nursing*, pp. 155–164. Maidenhead: Open University Press.

Smith, G (2014) *Mental Health Nursing at a Glance*. Chichester: Wiley Blackwell.

Smith, G. and Rylance, R. (2016) *Rapid Mental Health Nursing*. Chichester: Wiley Blackwell.

Smith, K.V. and Godfrey, N.S. (2002) Being a good nurse and doing the right thing: A qualitative study. *Nursing Ethics* 9(3): 301–312.

Smith Iltis, A. (2000) Bioethics as methodological case resolution: Specification, specified principlism and casuistry. *Journal of Medicine and Philosophy* 25(3): 271–284.

Strong, C. (2000) Specified principlism: What is it, and does it really resolve cases better than casuistry? *Journal of Medicine and Philosophy* 25 (3): 323–341.

Sumner, L.W. (1967) Normative ethics and metaethics. *Ethics* 77(2): 95–106.

Szasz, T.S. (1960) The myth of mental illness. *American Psychologist* 15(2): 113–118.

Thich Nhat Hanh (1995) *Peace is Every Step.* London: Rider.

Thornton, T. (2007) *Essential Philosophy of Psychiatry.* Oxford: Oxford University Press.

Tong, R. (2002) Teaching bioethics in the new millennium: Holding theories accountable to actual practices and real people. *Journal of Medicine and Philosophy* 27(4): 417–432.

Torrey, W.C., Drake, R.E., Dixon, L., Burns, B.J., Flynn, L., Rush, A.J., Clark, R.E. and Klatzker, D. (2001) Implementing evidence-based practices for persons with severe mental illnesses. *Psychiatric Services* 52(1): 45–50.

Tuijnman, A. and Bostrom, A. (2002) Changing notions of lifelong education and lifelong learning. *International Review of Education* 48(1/2): 93–110.

Varelius, J. (2009) Defining mental disorder in terms of our goals for demarcating mental disorder. *Philosophy, Psychiatry and Psychology* 16(1): 35–52.

Verkerk, M., Posltra, L. and de Jonge, M. (2008) Interference in psychiatric care: A sociological and ethical case analysis. In G. Widdershoven, J. MacMillan, J. Hope and L. Van der Scheer (eds), *Empirical Ethics in Psychiatry*, pp. 141–152. Oxford: Oxford University Press

Walsh, M. (2009) (Mis)representing mental distress? In J. Reynolds, R. Muston, T. Heller, J. Leach, M. McCormick, J. Wallcraft and M. Walsh (eds), *Mental Health Still Matters*, pp. 135–140. Basingstoke: Palgrave Macmillan.

Wand, T. (2011) Investigating the evidence for the effectiveness of risk assessment in mental health care. *Issues in Mental Health Nursing* 33(1): 2–7.

Watkins, J. (1998) *Hearing Voices: A Common Human Experience.* Melbourne: Hill of Content.

Watson, J.C. and Arp, R. (2011) *What's Good on TV? Understanding Ethics through Television.* Chichester: Wiley-Blackwell.

Welsh, I. and Lyons, C.M. (2001) Evidence-based care and the case for intuition and tacit knowledge in clinical assessment and decision making in mental health nursing practice: An empirical contribution to the debate. *Journal of Psychiatric and Mental Health Nursing* 8: 299–305.

Whitehead, B., Owen, P., Holmes, D., Beddingham, E., Simmons, M., Henshaw, L., Barton, M. and Walker, C. (2013) Supporting newly qualified nurses in the UK: A systematic literature review. *Nurse Education Today* 33(4): 370–377.

Wilkin, P. (2006) In search of the true self: a clinical journey through the vale of Soul-searching. *Journal of Psychiatric and Mental Health Nursing* 13: 12–18.

Wolff, J. (2006) *An Introduction To Political Philosophy* (rev. edn). Oxford: Oxford University Press.

Wolfs, C.A., de Vugt, M.E., Verkaaik, M., Haufe, M., Verkade, P.J., Verhey, F.R. and Stevens, F. (2012) Rational decision-making about treatment and care in dementia: A contradiction in terms? *Patient Education and Counseling* 87(1): 43–48.

Wong, E. (1997) *The Shambhala Guide to Taoism.* London: Shambhala.

Woodbridge, K. and Fulford, K.W.M. (2004) *Whose Values? A Workbook for Values-based Practice in Mental Health Care.* London: Sainsbury Centre for Mental Health.

Zande, M., Baart, A. and Vosman, F. (2014) Ethical sensitivity in practice: finding tacit moral knowing. *Journal of Advanced Nursing* 70(1): 68–76.

Zilboorg, G. and Henry, G.W. (1941) *A History of Medical Psychology.* London: George Allen & Unwin.

Legislation

Human Rights Act 1998: www.legislation.gov.uk/ukpga/1998/42/contents
Mental Capacity Act 2005: www.legislation.gov.uk/ukpga/2005/9/contents
Mental Health Act 1983: www.legislation.gov.uk/ukpga/1983/20/contents

INDEX